AF181311

The Successful Health Care Professional's Guide

Philip K. Louie • Michael H. McCarthy
Todd J. Albert
Editors

The Successful Health Care Professional's Guide

Everything You Need to Know But Weren't Taught in Training

Springer

Editors
Philip K. Louie
Center for Neurosciences and Spine
Virginia Mason Franciscan Health
Seattle, WA, USA

Michael H. McCarthy
Indiana Spine Group
University of Indiana
Carmel, IN, USA

Todd J. Albert
Department of Orthopaedic Surgery
Hospital for Special Surgery, Weill Cornell
Medical College
New York, NY, USA

ISBN 978-3-030-95949-4 ISBN 978-3-030-95950-0 (eBook)
https://doi.org/10.1007/978-3-030-95950-0

© The Editor(s) (if applicable) and The Author(s), under exclusive license to Springer Nature Switzerland AG 2022, corrected publication 2022
This work is subject to copyright. All rights are solely and exclusively licensed by the Publisher, whether the whole or part of the material is concerned, specifically the rights of translation, reprinting, reuse of illustrations, recitation, broadcasting, reproduction on microfilms or in any other physical way, and transmission or information storage and retrieval, electronic adaptation, computer software, or by similar or dissimilar methodology now known or hereafter developed.
The use of general descriptive names, registered names, trademarks, service marks, etc. in this publication does not imply, even in the absence of a specific statement, that such names are exempt from the relevant protective laws and regulations and therefore free for general use.
The publisher, the authors and the editors are safe to assume that the advice and information in this book are believed to be true and accurate at the date of publication. Neither the publisher nor the authors or the editors give a warranty, expressed or implied, with respect to the material contained herein or for any errors or omissions that may have been made. The publisher remains neutral with regard to jurisdictional claims in published maps and institutional affiliations.

This Springer imprint is published by the registered company Springer Nature Switzerland AG
The registered company address is: Gewerbestrasse 11, 6330 Cham, Switzerland

Louie: I dedicate this book to my wife Alice Louie, for her continued support throughout my training and career. To my parents, Douglas and Belinda, for their ongoing inspiration and belief. And to all my mentors, colleagues, and patients who provide me with the constant motivation to learn and educate.

McCarthy: To my wife Bridget, you are my everything.

Albert: To my daughter Emily and new son Bear, you have showed me the meaning and power of love, and how one partner can make another a better version of themselves.

The original version of this book was revised. The affiliation for book Editor Michael H. McCarthy has been updated. A correction to this chapter can be found at https://doi.org/10.1007/978-3-030-95950-0_15

Contents

Contributors

Noareen Zaheer Ahmed, MPH Office of Medical Leadership, Hospital for Special Surgery, New York, NY, USA

Todd J. Albert, MD Department of Orthopaedic Surgery, Hospital for Special Surgery, Weill Cornell Medical College, New York, NY, USA

Bryan Aristega Almeida Weill Cornell Medical College, Weill Cornell Medicine, New York, NY, USA

Alexandra Arguello Department of Orthopedic Surgery, Mayo Clinic, Rochester, MN, USA

William Cregar, MD Department of Orthopaedic Surgery, Rush University Medical Center, Chicago, IL, USA

James M. Dahle, MD, FACEP Department of Emergency Medicine, Jordan Valley Medical Center, West Jordan, UT, USA

Tobias Eng, CLU, ChFC, CFP Northwestern Mutual, Chicago, IL, USA

Karla J. Felix, PhD Hospital for Special Surgery, Academic Training, New York, NY, USA

Duretti Fufa, MD Hand and Upper Extremity Service, Hospital for Special Surgery, New York, NY, USA

Elizabeth Harry, MD, SFHM University of Colorado School of Medicine, UCHealth, Aurora, CO, USA

Alison M. Heru, MD Department of Psychiatry, University of Colorado Denver, Denver, CO, USA

Richard Joseph, MD, MBA Harvard Medical School, Brigham and Women's Hospital, Boston, MA, USA

Bryan T. Kelly, MD, MBA Office of Medical Leadership, Hospital for Special Surgery, New York, NY, USA

Jona Kerluku, BS Hand and Upper Extremity Service, Hospital for Special Surgery, New York, NY, USA

Darren Lee, MD, FRCPC Division of Physical Medicine and Rehabilitation, University of British Columbia, Vancouver, BC, Canada

Philip K. Louie, MD Center for Neurosciences and Spine, Virginia Mason Franciscan Health, Seattle, WA, USA

Michael H. McCarthy, MD, MPH Indiana Spine Group, University of Indiana, Carmel, IN, USA

Selina Poon Shriners Childrens Southern California, South Pasadena, CA, USA

Jesse Shen, MD Center for Neurosciences and Spine, Virginia Mason Franciscan Health, Seattle, WA, USA

Barbara Waxman, MS, MPA, PPC Odyssey Group Coaching LLC, San Francisco, CA, USA

Brandon Weiss, BS Lake Erie College of Osteopathic Medicine, Erie, PA, USA

Rick W. Wright Department of Orthopaedic Surgery, Vanderbilt University Medical Center, Nashville, TN, USA

Vijay Yanamadala, MD, MBA Hartford Healthcare, Westport, CT, USA

Quinnipiac University Frank H. Netter School of Medicine, North Haven, CT, USA

Introduction

1

Philip K. Louie, Michael H. McCarthy, and Todd J. Albert

Healthcare education and training are facing major crossroads right now. Over the past few years, we have witnessed various attempts at redesigning and pivoting chunks of curriculum. The long-standing notion of providing almost exclusive education and training based on specialty-specific content is slowly shifting. In our opinion, has done an excellent job in providing all the content-related knowledge within specific specialties. However, training on how to effectively integrate this knowledge and various skills across previously built silos, and encourage continued collaboration that ultimately grows and innovates, is lacking.

For many, this period of education/training is during formative years of early adulthood. Many of the skill sets described this book are often overlooked in the traditional curriculum. Yet, recent graduates are expected to understand and utilize these skills immediately upon graduation (and entering the "real world").

There are numerous texts available that provide content and career-based aids and teaching materials for students pursuing a career in a healthcare profession. These previous publications often target students and trainees at specific intervals of training, that focus on their specific specialty. These are important texts that provide valuable information that support the students/trainees through their season of training and can provide essential materials to learn the necessary content and guide skills training. As long as we can remember, many of these texts are considered the backbone to education and training.

P. K. Louie (✉)
Center for Neurosciences and Spine, Virginia Mason Franciscan Health, Seattle, WA, USA
e-mail: philip.louie@virginiamason.org

M. H. McCarthy
Indiana Spine Group, University of Indiana, Carmel, IN, USA

T. J. Albert
Department of Orthopaedic Surgery, Hospital for Special Surgery, Weill Cornell Medical College, New York, NY, USA

© The Author(s), under exclusive license to Springer Nature Switzerland AG 2022, corrected publication 2022

P. K. Louie et al. (eds.), *The Successful Health Care Professional's Guide*,
https://doi.org/10.1007/978-3-030-95950-0_1

Often overlooked, there are many aspects of the education and training process and continuing education that are critical to excel at any stage, and to thrive at the level of the end goal. The subject of specialty specific training is incredibly important and will always be a critical focus. However, we believe that certain skills and principles are essential in reaching peak performance during training, career, and life. Topics including leadership, goal-setting, mentorship, relationships, skills-training (outside perspective), stoicism, financial planning are among the many topics that are critical in healthcare-career development, but require searching through numerous resources to learn. Training for any healthcare profession is already difficult and fraught with long hours trying to learn endless material and skills.

The goal of this book is to provide a comprehensive resource of various "essential" skills and practices that have been previously overlooked in many traditional training curriculae. As having completed the rigorous training involved in these professions, we understand the value of take-home points for each topic. Key points and tangible action items will be provided for each section, geared specifically to you, the learner! Although focused for the healthcare profession, authors from various sectors and professional backgrounds have dedicated their time and efforts to contribute their expertise to this collection.

Perseverance and Grit: Tools for a Successful Career in Healthcare

2

Karla J. Felix and Jona Kerluku

Introduction

Admissions committees use several metrics of information to make decisions on inviting applicants for an interview to competitive healthcare professional programs [2]. It is not only academics, leadership experience, research, or past work experiences that are taken into consideration by selection committees. More recently, institutions look for candidates that can articulate ability to overcome obstacles and evidence of perseverance, with the latter shown to be an independent predictor of success [3, 4]. Desire, overcome obstacles, relentless, stamina, devotion, never stop, proactive leader and tireless worker--these are the words that stand out after reading hundreds of applications to a competitive healthcare professional program. These are also the words that are synonymous with grit, defined by Angela Duckworth in 2007 as "passion and perseverance for long-term goals" [1].

In deconstructing grit for students pursuing a career in healthcare, one can find that these candidates have a passion for helping people. This passion is often demonstrated through overcoming a personal illness or maybe navigating their loved one's ability to obtain adequate healthcare, leading them toward a quest to remedy that for others. This passion for helping people contributes to a narrow focus and a deep need to meet that purpose. It is the perseverance through hardships or discouragements in their life that allows the most successful students to never give up and exude resiliency. Healthcare professions are especially challenging for the rigorous lengthy training, therefore students interested in this career path are known to have

K. J. Felix (✉)
Hospital for Special Surgery, Academic Training, New York, NY, USA
e-mail: felixk@hss.edu

J. Kerluku
Hand and Upper Extremity Service, Hospital for Special Surgery, New York, NY, USA
e-mail: kerlukuj@hss.edu

© The Author(s), under exclusive license to Springer Nature Switzerland AG 2022

P. K. Louie et al. (eds.), *The Successful Health Care Professional's Guide*,
https://doi.org/10.1007/978-3-030-95950-0_2

long-term goals, which often include developing improved health care models, curiosity to create novel delivery of care or deep commitments to helping undeserved communities.

However, getting your feet firmly planted in the healthcare field requires a level of grit that sets you apart from the average population. Skills associated with motivation and attitude, termed noncognitive traits, were historically considered important for athletics and/or military and have only recently been studied throughout the health professions. Grit in particular is often interchanged with resilience, although these are different concepts [7, 8]. Grit is defined as "applying passion and sustained persistence toward long-term achievement, with no particular concern for rewards or recognition along the way" [21]. Resilience, alternatively, is "demonstrating the ability to recover from or adjust easily to misfortune or change" [21]. Since proposed by Duckworth in 2007, scientists have more recently taken an interest in better understanding how grit contributes to a learner's performance and achievement.

Limited research has associated high grit and resilience scores from students in multiple healthcare specialties, including nursing, pharmacy, and medical students, to greater course engagement, improved self-reflection, and overall high academic performance [24]. One of the early studies on grit in the medical student population came out of a simple question: what is the difference in grit between medical students compared to residents, who are more advanced in their medical training? With orthopaedic surgery currently being one of the most competitive medical specialties, this subspecialty served as a viable population to assess grit. This study compared the use of noncognitive/personality variables for the future possibility of selecting medical students into orthopaedic residency [5]. Measures of self-control, conscientiousness and grit in addition to the standard cognitive measures of selection were examined. Conscientiousness is a similar quality to grit, but what sets the construct apart is that grit encompasses behavior that showcases the discipline and diligence to pursue a targeted goal, sometimes when obstacles are present. This study revealed that there are common personality traits among those completing a post-graduate medical education – grit, self-control and conscientiousness. While there were similar levels of both conscientiousness and self-control, there were increased levels of grit displayed by medical students applying to residency [5].

Naturally, the follow up question now is: do these grit levels change from residency to independent medical practice? In a longitudinal study of over 2000 attending orthopaedic surgeons and over 800 residency applicants, it was found that both attending surgeons and orthopaedic residents possessed similar levels of grit higher than the general population [20]. Grit is a successful predictor of sustained effort and achievement in many circumstances, but as the literature shows, grit scores echoed the degree of sustained drive that the trainees have to succeed. Other healthcare professions, such as nursing and pharmacy, are beginning to prioritize investigating grit over resiliency to clarify how grit plays a role in overcoming the multiple challenges presented during training and beyond.

Can Grit Be Taught?

The predictive role of grit in academic achievement yields several studies with similar findings suggesting that grittier individuals attain higher levels of education and make fewer career transitions [1]. Grit has long lasting effects in one's professional trajectory, especially in healthcare. Having grit will pull trainees through the long hours, the academic and administrative demands as well as the transitions in life (i.e., getting married, having children). With the high rates of empirical research on grit and its relationship with academic success, [2–6, 9–14, 19–21, 24], few studies have examined the relationship between other factors associated with grit and overall success in the profession. One such study, uniquely identified observable practice activities (OPA) to assess noncognitive skills in the practice setting so that educators can use it for formative and summative assessment [21]. An OPA is a "discrete work-based assessment of elements collected over time and mapped to larger structures such as milestones, entrustable professional activities, or competencies" [21]. The OPAs identified were characterized by eighteen noncognitive attributes, one of which is grit (Table 2.1). Clarifying the observable behaviors that showcase grit can help guide learners while also helping educators provide feedback throughout training. The authors caution that it is not enough to report back to the student on the attribute but to give concrete examples of such attributes (i.e., OPAs) and that institutions should factor in external or contextual elements too that may interfere or promote such attributes.

Table 2.1 Observable behaviors that demonstrate grit, a growth mindset, and resilience

Characteristic:	Demonstrating observable behaviors[a]:
Grit	Answering questions even if wrong on prior responses Continuing to work despite setbacks and failures Remains committed to quality patient care even during stressful clinical shifts Capable of identifying valuable learning opportunities even throughout routine work tasks Sets ambitious goals after failures
Growth mindset	Seeks immediate feedback to assess areas of improvement Able to implement goals for improvement after self-assessment using test results or other performance data Helps others in their journey of self-improvement and growth
Resilience	Habitually reflects and debriefs with mentors or peers on challenging experiences Actively learns from mistakes to optimize outcomes Responds with positive attitude even after negative feedback or poor exam scores Agile and does not dwell, able to quickly recover from small failures Proactively uses negative systemic experiences to improve working and learning environments

[a]Adapted from Warm et al. [21]

How Do You Measure Your Grit?

Grit has a valid, tested measurement tool that was first studied and implemented by Angela Duckworth [1] in several populations from middle school children to West Point Academy cadets. As the survey tool took flights, it was only natural that researchers would eventually study the health professions as these careers are known for employing self-reported resilient individuals [25]. Often in the literature, researchers use the short grit scale (SGS) in addition to demographic and personal information. The SGS includes high grit (positive) and low grit (negative) related questions on a 5-point scale, with higher numbers indicating more grit. Dr. Duckworth published the 8-item scale on her website, making it easily accessible to anyone curious to learn about the questions.

Try taking the test yourself now (Fig. 2.1) to measure your grit using the scoring guide below (Fig. 2.2) to briefly evaluate how passionate and persevering you see yourself to be.

Test Your Grit!

Directions for taking the Grit Scale [22, 23]: Here are a number of statements that may or may not apply to you. For the most accurate score, when responding, think of how you compare to most people not just the people you know well, but most people in the world. There are no right or wrong answers, so just answer honestly.

Can Grit Protect Medical Trainees From Burnout?

The demands of the healthcare professions lead to many findings of increased rates of burnout [25, 26]. Emotional exhaustion, cynicism and/or perception of professional accomplishments being reduced are characteristics of burnout. Burnout is often measured by a validated Maslach Burnout Inventory (MBI) and particularly MBI- Student Survey is used with medical students [16]. The survey consists of three different subscales: Emotional Exhaustion, Cynicism and Personal Inefficacy. High scores on the survey indicate burnout. Generally, burnout is a consequence of workplace stress [15, 16] but also associated with high demands in medical training learning environments that involve intense competition among classmates and heavy cognitive load [17, 18].

Medical trainees are at risk for burnout at any professional career stage, causing risk for increased medical errors, suicidal ideation, substance abuse and relationship difficulties.

Generally, when entering medical school, students have lower burnout rates, are less depressed, and report higher quality of life. However, as early as completing their first year of medical school, students are at risk for experiencing above average

Short Grit Scale

1. New ideas and projects sometimes distract me from previous ones.

- ☐ Very much like me.
- ☐ Mostly like me.
- ☐ Somewhat like me.
- ☐ Not much like me.
- ☐ Not like me at all.

2. Setbacks don't discourage me. I don't give up easily.

- ☐ Very much like me.
- ☐ Mostly like me.
- ☐ Somewhat like me.
- ☐ Not much like me.
- ☐ Not like me at all.

3. I often set a goal but later choose to pursue a different one.

- ☐ Very much like me.
- ☐ Mostly like me.
- ☐ Somewhat like me.
- ☐ Not much like me.
- ☐ Not like me at all.

4. I am a hard worker.

- ☐ Very much like me.
- ☐ Mostly like me.
- ☐ Somewhat like me.
- ☐ Not much like me.
- ☐ Not like me at all.

5. I have difficulty maintaining my focus on projects that take more than a few months to complete.

- ☐ Very much like me.
- ☐ Mostly like me.
- ☐ Somewhat like me.
- ☐ Not much like me.
- ☐ Not like me at all.

6. I finish whatever I begin.

- ☐ Very much like me.
- ☐ Mostly like me.
- ☐ Somewhat like me.
- ☐ Not much like me.
- ☐ Not like me at all.

7. I am diligent. I never give up.

- ☐ Very much like me.
- ☐ Mostly like me.
- ☐ Somewhat like me.
- ☐ Not much like me.
- ☐ Not like me at all.

8. I have been obsessed with a certain idea or project for a short time but later lost interest.

- ☐ Very much like me.
- ☐ Mostly like me.
- ☐ Somewhat like me.
- ☐ Not much like me.
- ☐ Not like me at all.

Fig. 2.1 Short 8-Item Grit Scale

burnout rates [17, 18, 25–27]. After evaluating student traits such as tolerance for ambiguity, grit, religiosity, and social support, studies found that grittier students had lower burnout scores (measured by the MBI- Student Survey) after one year of medical school. All other variables measured either had no correlation with burnout or were not shown to have a protective effect against burnout [26]. Other studies have consistently shown that grit scores increase with increasing age suggesting that experience obtained throughout medical training and progressions in the career help to prevent burnout.

Scoring Guide: Add up all the points and divide by 8.

For questions 2, 4, 7, and 8 assign the following points.

5 = Very much like me
4 = Mostly like me
3 = Somewhat like me
2 = Not much like me
1 = Not like me at all

For questions 1, 3, 5, and 6 assign the following points.

1 = Very much like me
2 = Mostly like me
3 = Somewhat like me
4 = Not much like me
5 = Not like me at all

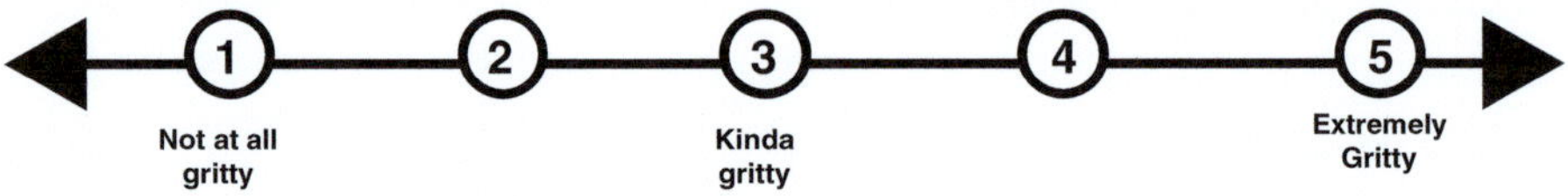

Fig. 2.2 Scoring Guide and Relative Grit Performance

Tips on How to Get Grittier

Studies show that grit can be taught, although standardized evidence-based strategies are still being developed [1, 10, 29–31]. Here are four signs that you already possess grit, no matter how you scored on the short grit scale [28].

1. There are things you already find fascinating.
2. You view mistakes as a normal part of the process.
3. You consistently attempt to make work more meaningful.
4. You are hopeful that you can change and grow.

You can improve your grit scores by working on the following aspects:

1. ***Pursue what interests you.***

If you chose to complete the rigorous training required to succeed in a healthcare profession, chances are that it already interests you. Further decision making is often presented to nursing and medical students when it comes to choosing a specialty. When deciding, it would benefit you to first make sure you "fall in love with something" as Angela Duckworth says [31]. It is not enough to just reflect on experiences, since that work is centered on moments that have already happened. You need to also be open to exploring several new potential interests or even revisiting old interests to figure out what feels best for you and your career.

2. ***Deliberate practice on improving weaknesses.***

While exploring these interests, one must develop a capacity for doing hard work [31]. It can feel discouraging to get answers wrong, score poorly on practice exams, or feel like you may not know enough during clinical rotations. However, look for opportunities to get feedback from mentors or your peers. We are more likely to follow through when we are good at something, and the best way to get good at a skill is through practice. First, identify your strengths to help you gain confidence. The next part, where you need to be most honest with yourself, is figuring out what areas you could improve on. You can do this by using objective data reports, such as test scores or rotation evaluations. However, you do not need to tackle this process alone. Try asking for feedback directly from peers and mentors who have seen your work ethic (see more in other chapters about how to do this effectively). Then, make sure you set specific, measurable goals to address your weaknesses. Dedicating time on your calendar to make sure you complete these action items will help you stay consistent and allow you to better measure progress.

3. ***Find your purpose.***

Having a clear concise answer of your life purpose has been shown to lead to up upward spiral of motivation, benefiting not only for your career but areas of your personal life as well [31]. We spoke about healthcare workers entering their chosen profession because they are dedicated to helping others. However, clarifying what exactly what you do that helps others will guide you to finding your purpose. Helping patients through some of their most vulnerable moments is extremely fulfilling work that you may supplement with research or mentoring. Spend some time deeply reflecting, and journaling about what your core values are and how the work you do or want to do connects to those values in meaningful ways.

4. ***Be hopeful.***

Hope is hard to measure scientifically. But we know how we feel when we have it, and when we don't. Angela Duckworth says that "grit depends on a different kind of hope" [31]. She explains that rather than passively asking for the universe to improve our circumstances, the gritty hope has nothing to do with serendipity. The hope you need if you want to improve your grit levels is believing that your effort and direct actions can improve your future outcomes. Research has attempted to track this emotion by evaluating our motivational systems and found that when people lack hope, they tend to gravitate toward easier unchallenging tasks and tend to not feel in control of their environment [32]. A growth-mindset can help actively reestablish hope in addition to incorporating more optimistic self-talk [31]. Just changing our attitude to highlight efforts, strategies, and choices over outcomes, and more positively reacting to failure can bring hope back into your life, and in turn help you develop grit. You can achieve what you want only if you believe you can first.

5. ***Spend more time other gritty people.***

Quality healthcare depends on the collaboration and clear communication from several units. In this way, there is a special opportunity to directly network with professionals within your field and find those who you think exhibit the level of grit you want to have. Forming strong connections with colleagues and peers across many areas of healthcare will not only broaden your perspectives, but it might open you up to new possibilities to fulfill your purpose. Even if you are not actively seeking new job opportunities, networking is still a useful strategy that will benefit your career long-term. Strategies to build stronger relationships could be staying in touch with former colleagues or setting a goal to make a certain number of new connections for a given time period. You most certainly do not need to stay only within your specialty when meeting new people. Try leveraging social media to connect with other healthcare professionals or industries. Some productive collaborations could include developing new research studies, internal institutional initiatives with colleagues, or broader activism work. In time you will find that the norms and values of others, in addition to their work ethic, will soon blend into your own.

Conclusion

A common theme across the literature revealed that the domain of grit should be objectively considered for application review committees in academic institutions and job positions. Grit can be used as a tool to holistically evaluate individuals and could be weighed equally to common academic factors such as test scores and volunteer work. Since grit in an individual is defined as being deeply passionate about something that provides intrinsic meaning, this trait is credited to helping students navigate challenges in the long and arduous road to becoming a healthcare professional. As the literature suggests, students with high grit are more likely to complete successful training throughout their healthcare career. There is promise that grit can be taught and practiced for each career stage.

References

1. Duckworth AL, Peterson C, Matthews MD, Kelly DR. Grit: perseverance and passion for long-term goals. J Pers Soc Psychol. 2007;92(6):1087–101. https://doi.org/10.1037/0022-3514.92.6.1087.
2. Brothers TE, Wetherholt S. Importance of the faculty interview during the resident application process. J Surg Educ. 2007; https://doi.org/10.1016/j.jsurg.2007.05.003.
3. Shih AF, Maroongroge S. The importance of grit in medical training. J Grad Med Educ. 2017;9(3):399. https://doi.org/10.4300/JGME-D-16-00852.1.
4. Ray R, Brown J. Reassessing student potential for medical school success: distance traveled, grit, and hardiness. Mil Med. 2015;180(4):138–41.
5. Kelly AM, Townsend KW, Davis S, Nouryan L, Bostrom MP, Felix KJ. Comparative assessment of grit, conscientiousness, and self-control in applicants interviewing for residency positions and current orthopaedic surgery residents. J Surg Educ. 2017;75:557.
6. Bazelais P, et al. Grit, mindset, and academic performance: a study of pre-university science students. Eurasia J Math Sci Technol Educ. 2018;14(12):em1615. https://doi.org/10.29333/ejmste/94570
7. Eskreis-Winkler L, Shulman EP, Beal SA, Duckworth AL. The grit effect: predicting retention in the military, the workplace, school and marriage. Front Psychol. 2014;5(FEB):36. https://doi.org/10.3389/fpsyg.2014.00036.
8. Seligman MEP. GRIT, character, and achievement: a new theory of intelligence. In: Flourish: a visionary new understanding of happiness and well-being. New York: Free; 2011. N. pag. Print.

9. Christopoulou M, et al. The role of grit in education: a systematic review. Psychology. 2018;9(15):2951–71.
10. Credé M, Tynan MC, Harms PD. Much ado about grit: a meta-analytic synthesis of the grit literature. J Pers Soc Psychol. 2017;113(3):492.
11. Fernández-Martín FD, Arco-Tirado JL, Hervás-Torres M. Grit as a predictor and outcome of educational, professional, and personal success: a systematic review. Educ Psychol. 2020;26(2):163–73.
12. Miller-Matero LR, Martinez S, MacLean L, Yaremchuk K, Ko AB. Grit: a predictor of medical student performance. Educ Health (Abingdon). 2018;31(2):109–13. https://doi.org/10.4103/efh.EfH_152_16.
13. Jumat MR, Chow PKH, Allen JC, et al. Grit protects medical students from burnout: a longitudinal study. BMC Med Educ. 2020;20:266. https://doi.org/10.1186/s12909-020-02187-1
14. Isenberg G, Brown A, DeSantis J, Veloski J, Hojat M. The relationship between grit and selected personality measures in medical students. Int J Med Educ. 2020;11:25–30. Published 2020 Jan 30. https://doi.org/10.5116/ijme.5e01.f32d.
15. WHO WHO. ICD-11 for mortality and morbidity statistics (Vervion 04/19). 2019.
16. Maslach C, Jackson SE, Leiter MP. Maslach burnout inventory manual. Palo Alto, CA: Consulting Psychologists Press; 1996.
17. Santen SA, Holt DB, Kemp JD, Hemphill RR. Burnout in medical students: examining the prevalence and associated factors. South Med J. 2010;103(8):758–63. 22.
18. Dyrbye LN, Thomas MR, Harper W, Massie FS Jr, Power DV, Eacker A, et al. The learning environment and medical student burnout: a multicentre study. Med Educ. 2009;43(3):274–82.
19. Welch JC. Assessing grit and conscientiousness to predict medical student success on the National USMLE Step 2 Clinical Knowledge Exam, 2020. Dissertations - ALL. 1286. https://surface.syr.edu/etd/1286
20. Samuelsen BT, Desai VS, Turner NS, Kelly AM, Grawe B, Camp CL. Generational differences in grit, self-control, and conscientiousness among orthopaedic surgeons: from millennials to baby boomers. J Bone Joint Surg Am. 2019;101(14):e71. https://doi.org/10.2106/JBJS.18.00275.
21. Warm EJ, Kinnear B, Lance S, Schauer DP, Brenner J. What behaviors define a good physician? Assessing and communicating about noncognitive skills [published online ahead of print, 2021 Jun 22]. Acad Med. 2021; https://doi.org/10.1097/ACM.0000000000004215.
22. Duckworth AL, Quinn PD. Development and validation of the short grit scale (Grit-S). J Pers Assess. 2009;91(2):166–74. https://doi.org/10.1080/00223890802634290.
23. Duckworth AL, Peterson C, Matthews MD, Kelly DR. Grit: perseverance and passion for long-term goals. J Pers Soc Psychol. 2007;9:1087–101.
24. Stoffel JM, Cain J. Review of grit and resilience literature within health professions education. Am J Pharm Educ. 2018;82(2):6150. https://doi.org/10.5688/ajpe6150.
25. Halliday L, Walker A, Vig S, Hines J, Brecknell J. Grit and burnout in UK doctors: a cross-sectional study across specialties and stages of training. Postgrad Med J. 2017;93(1101):389–94. https://doi.org/10.1136/postgradmedj-2015-133919.
26. Bridgeman PJ, Bridgeman MB, Barone J. Burnout syndrome among healthcare professionals. Am J Health Syst Pharm. 2018;75(3):147–52. https://doi.org/10.2146/ajhp170460.
27. Jumat MR, Chow PK, Allen JC Jr, et al. Grit protects medical students from burnout: a longitudinal study. BMC Med Educ. 2020;20(1):266. Published 2020 Aug 12. https://doi.org/10.1186/s12909-020-02187-1.
28. Hilmantel R. 4 Signs you have grit. 2016, May 12. https://time.com/4327035/4-signs-you-have-grit/
29. Calo M, Peiris C, Chipchase L, Blackstock F, Judd B. Grit, resilience and mindset in health students. Clin Teach. 2019;16(4):317–22. https://doi.org/10.1111/tct.13056.
30. Dweck CS. Mindset: the new psychology of success. Random House; 2006.
31. Duckworth A. Grit: the power of passion and perseverance. 1st ed. Scribner Book Company; 2016.
32. Kaufman S. Ungifted: intelligence redefined. 1st ed. Basic Books; 2013.

What We Can Learn from Artistic and Athletic Disciplines about Skills Training

3

Jesse Shen, Darren Lee, and William Cregar

What We Can Learn from Music

Technical Aspects of Practice and Improvement

Music is an artistic endeavor that is highly technical. No musician can perform at the highest level without brilliant technical skills. How do musicians train to acquire technical proficiency? The process of skill acquisition can be broken down to a granular level, and this can ultimately be something that we as clinicians can learn.

The adage that practice makes perfect can be misleading. As many musicians agree, only perfect practice makes perfect. Perfect practice can easily parallel to proceduralists in medicine in that practicing in an inefficient way will only lead to an ineffective practice.

Musicians all usually follow a standard workflow to acquire perfection for a new instrument or musical piece. As I was told during my training as a pianist, you need to start playing a part slowly, but it must be perfectly played with crisp technique. Once technical proficiency is obtained, the tempo is then increased progressively until the desired level. The idea behind this slow, deliberate learning method is that it reinforces proper coordination and muscle memory to a passage that will translate into greater speed with excellent technical proficiency.

In contrast, when musicians practice a musical piece too quickly before technical mastery, it leads to sloppy, inefficient, and poor quality of music. The problem with this approach is that it overlooks the acquisition of technical proficiency and

J. Shen
Center for Neurosciences and Spine, Virginia Mason Franciscan Health, Seattle, WA, USA

D. Lee (✉)
Division of Physical Medicine and Rehabilitation, University of British Columbia, Vancouver, BC, Canada

W. Cregar
Department of Orthopaedic Surgery, Rush University Medical Center, Chicago, IL, USA

© The Author(s), under exclusive license to Springer Nature Switzerland AG 2022

P. K. Louie et al. (eds.), *The Successful Health Care Professional's Guide*,
https://doi.org/10.1007/978-3-030-95950-0_3

ultimately reinforces terrible habits that can be challenging to correct. This problem parallels multiple facets of medicine, not only in surgical specialties where the link is obvious but in medical specialties where completeness and systematic approaches to histories or physical exams are needed before increasing efficiency.

Often acquisition of skills can be daunting. Some aspects are more challenging than others, and sometimes we simply don't know where to start. Similarly, breaking down an entire piece of music into manageable smaller tasks or passages to work on can help us advance towards our goals. This breakdown can also help us reflect and identify areas of improvement. For example, playing a technical piece such as Chopin's Op.53 in A flat major (Polonaise) may require practicing the more challenging passages rather than the entire piece repeatedly. All these smaller tasks or passages will be mastered gradually, and putting them all together will produce a masterpiece.

In parallel, an aspiring surgeon may need to break down some complex techniques into smaller tasks to acquire these skills progressively. No surgeon will immediately perform a three-column osteotomy of the spine on their first day of residency. Skills require gradual work of smaller tasks and practice of more challenging aspects to become competent and safe.

Finally, as we have touched on, self-reflection is an essential component of practice and improvement. Musicians will often review recordings, previous performances and even film themselves practicing identifying potential areas of improvement. This self-reflection is of critical importance as it is particularly true in medicine. Having peers around you to ask for counsel or even review a past case to see what areas can be improved is vital for a surgeon. Furthermore, we as physicians must develop reflexes to continuously improve our practice for the next patient under our care. This mindset of self-reflection will ultimately benefit the patient.

Goals and Performance of Music

What are the goals of the individual musician? Is it to be a solo performer at a jazz café or be part of a philharmonic orchestra? Our personal goals will ultimately help decide how best to practice, what mentors to seek and what tours or venues to play in. Having a vision and focus of the future is as essential for a musician as a physician.

Do you want a private practice or academic career? Do you want to be a subspecialist or generalist? These questions are critical not only early in training but are continuously re-evaluated during a career. It is important to define goals and provide focus to invest your energies.

However, your career, much like performing music, may change throughout time. Your style, approach, and technical abilities will evolve, and it is important to embrace them. David Grohl started as a drummer for Nirvana and eventually developed a successful career as a guitarist and singer for the Foo Fighters later in his career. Your goals may shift throughout time, and it is essential to recognize them. Your focus and energy towards your vision will ultimately lead you to become that person.

Once the goals have been set, the practice invested, it is time to perform. The context of the performance is incredibly varied in music. Musicians can have many roles, either being a soloist, band member, or orchestra member. Each of these roles has different responsibilities and needs the right sets of skills.

Like an orchestra, healthcare is a greater sum of all the moving parts within it. The conductor, the wind instruments, strings, percussion all work in the same flow to create beautiful music. Everyone involved must be attentive and respectful of others. The flow of the group is more important than the individual, and this is a common characteristic between orchestral music and healthcare delivery. A surgeon may thus need to be mindful of the music he decides to play in the operating room. It may increase their workflow and even their performance but may hinder others [1].

Ultimately, performing music is an art. There will always be a set of rules or tempo and notes that need to be sharp or flat. But the musician plays to his style and interpretation of a musical piece. Medicine is similar as there is an art to its practice. How do you approach informed consent with your patients? How do you approach a terminally ill patient and their family? There is an artistic side to medicine, and each physician has their style and approach. Understanding how you perform in medicine and the practice necessary to get there will enhance your skills.

Balance Between Music and Life

Like sports and medicine, performing music requires the musician to be at peak performance [2]. This state of achieving excellent and consistent results is an essential aspect of the performing arts. However, this requires balance. The balance between the practice to strive for excellence and the rest to maintain health and mental acuity.

This balance means that good nutrition, sleep, and time away from music are just as important as the practice that goes into technical brilliance, as discussed previously. Consistent achievement of results needs consistent state of physical, mental, and emotional states. This balance is critical for personal growth within music as well as the professional lives of physicians.

This balance is especially important in the context that there's always more to learn. The learning never ends. This lifelong learning is true for musicians as techniques can always be sharpened further, and new musical pieces require a new set of skills. Styles can change as the trends in music are always changing. Being a lifelong learner is also true for medicine, and having the right balance will continue improving. Having the right balance allows us to grow and keep growing towards our ultimate goals no matter what they are.

Balance also means having the right people surround you in life. Family, friends, and colleagues, inspiration, and support come from all around us. Mentors can be beneficial as they can often continue to provide guidance even outside of traditional teachings, such as in our lives and our careers. Advice is always welcomed, and an outside pair of eyes can give us perspective on balancing it all. Table 3.1 summarizes the take home points from this section of the chapter.

Table 3.1 Summary of recommendations from what can be learned from music

What we can learn from music	Practical recommendations
Perfect practice	When learning a new technique, always start slow and progressively increase speed
Work and life balance	Schedule time for physical activity
	Prioritize sleep
Creating goals	List milestones that are measurable and a timeframe for each of them

Table 3.2 Summary of recommendations from what can be learned from sports

What we can learn from sports	Recommendations
Preparation	Visualize and write down detailed steps of a procedure or patient encounter
	Practice skills or acquire knowledge outside of hospital and work hours to enhance progression
Perseverance	Identify a mentor that can guide you towards your goals
	Critique your work and list areas of potential improvement everyday
Passion	Define your purpose and write it down as a constant reminder

What We Can Learn from Sports

Similar to music, many training techniques from sports can be translated into medical training (Table 3.2). Preparation off the field is vital for peak performance on the field. This section of the chapter continues the discussion of what we can learn from music, but with sports as an inspiration for skills acquisition in medicine.

Preparation

Sports is often defined by moments, and some performances can be fleeting moments. As an example, the 100-meter sprint at the Olympics is won in under 10 seconds. However, it doesn't reflect the preparation and the time it took to achieve such performance.

We have previously discussed how perfect practice makes perfect. This concept of perfect practice also holds for sports as this dedication to perfection is effectively produced through practice. This concept is an essential component of medicine as the training is not limited to the confines of the hospital. But it also is practiced off the "medical field." An example would be the surgeon continuously using his non-dominant hand in his daily life to enhance bi-manual dexterity.

Visualization is another crucial part of the preparation that makes successful athletes and physicians, and this holds especially true for surgeons [3, 4]. Visualizing how a race or how a surgical procedure will flow is an essential component of developing skills and the ability to anticipate potential problems during a performance, either in sports or surgery. This visualization allows us to anticipate each step without even holding an instrument, ultimately refining our technique and workflow.

Knowing where each instrument needs to go and when to call for help in a potential crisis are all helpful to improve our techniques and efficiency.

This visualization can also be applied to practice as, famously, Michael Phelps' coach would sabotage him during practice, or small swim meets to be prepared for when it could potentially happen in a big event. Although this cannot be performed in a clinical setting for obvious ethical reasons in medicine, always having more than one plan in the management of patients can be a good visualization routine. Visualization also allows the physician to be prepared during surgery and avoids being caught off guard when an issue arises.

Similar to visualization, observing masters of the discipline is also a component that allows us to develop skills both on the track and in the operating room. Observing the strokes of Olympic champions can pay dividends for the aspiring swimmer by attempting to replicate these champions. Similarly, watching a master surgeon and paying attention to the minute details such as retractor positioning allows the junior surgeon to improve efficiency and technical skill.

Preparation is also part of your everyday life. Nathan Mackinnon, an all-star ice hockey centerman, was described by his teammate as being one of the most prepared athletes. Every aspect of his life was geared towards peak performance in hockey. He would have a personal chef cook all his meals geared towards hockey. He also has a personal physical trainer and physical therapist dedicated to improving his performance. Surgeons have been compared to elite athletes [5] and this attitude that your daily habits are part of your preparation in the medical field holds.

Perseverance

Perseverance and resilience are vital components in skill acquisition and achieving peak performance. Perseverance is critical for high-performance athletes as a career is often filled with disappointments and failures. Michael Jordan was famously cut from his high school basketball team. Imagine if this failure had stopped him from becoming a six-time NBA champion. Acquiring a new skill, whatever it might be, will be associated with failure. But these failures often are our greatest teachers and will show us avenues of improvement. Learning how to fail and surmounting these failures will ultimately allow us to improve.

Most skills require teachers, and in sports, it requires good coaches. Coaches are usually mentors as well as teachers for both athletes and physicians. Being coachable is an expression that is commonly used in sports, and it applies equally in medicine. Being coachable encompasses not only perseverance but also work ethic and the ability to use constructive criticism as a learning opportunity to improve. Indeed, this also takes good coaches such as Phil Jackson as he coached Michael Jordan to 6 NBA championships.

Being coachable also means that you need the ability to self-critique and be honest with yourself. The objective in sports is often straightforward. How fast did you run or swim? The evidence is clear on how you performed. However, it is much more difficult in medicine as the objectives are often unclear or the milestones are not defined. Having a good coach and mentor is thus critical in addition to having clear goals in training.

Finally, adaptation plays hand in hand with perseverance. In sports, this is often highlighted by athletes aging or needing to adapt their game due to other factors such as injuries. Furthermore, sometimes the game itself changes, such as the sweeping new rule changes in the NHL after 2005 that made the game much faster than before. The physician can learn from sports that adaption is a continuous process throughout one's career and even in developing skills. After formal residency or fellowship training, the adaption continues throughout one's practice. As technology continues to change and impact our practice, adaptability remains vital if one wants to stay "on top of their game" or run the risk of becoming a dinosaur.

Motivation and Passion

Passion is not specific to the sporting world, but it is undoubtedly an easy example. Would Tom Brady still be chasing another Superbowl after being a seven-time champion at the age of 44 without passion? Would Roger Federer be chasing another Wimbledon Championship at 40 without passion? Passion is also a driver in medicine, and it is one of the drivers of the pursuit of excellence in patient care. This driver is a passion that motivates us to practice, visualize and continuously push ourselves to become better every day.

Our passion stems from the reason we do what we do. In sports, aiming to become the GOAT (greatest of all time) in tennis or striving to become the fastest man on land are some clear examples that are quantifiable. The drive to succeed in achieving the goals and the work necessary to achieve them becomes apparent.

The same can be said about medicine and even in training. By defining the reason for why we do things, like how Simon Sinek beautifully described in his seminal TedTalk, is what will ultimately drive us and fuel our passion. From there, defining our objectives will become a roadmap to channel our energy and passion.

Setting goals is critical in the pursuit of success as it channels our focus with clear milestones. Our time frames can define objectives. What objective have we defined for today? This month? This year or this decade? Having these goals set allows us to be kept on track in a world where distraction is seemingly everywhere. Setting goals based on time frames also will enable us to develop a roadmap with our mentors and coaches.

This concept of goal setting is easy to translate in a surgical setting. In training, setting goals for an operative day and what objectives you want to attain from a rotation can be quickly drawn out after careful thought. Creating well-defined tangible goals will ultimately create a clear roadmap to growth, improvement, and success in surgery.

Final Thoughts

Many elements from music and sports can be inspired in the training of a physician. The quality of practice, the ethics in work, and resilience are all key elements that make elite athletes or successful musicians. The physician can inspire these traits in developing skills and achieving career goals.

Being mindful of what we want to achieve is critically important in our professional careers. Mindfulness and introspection allow us to set goals both in the short and long term. This mindfulness will enable us to channel our energies in a focused and oriented manner. Having clear objectives and a passion for achieving them will also allow our mentors and teachers to push us towards those goals.

Hopefully, this chapter provides the reader some food for thought and introspection on how we as physicians can become better. Acquiring new skills and competency is a lifelong process that will inevitably have its challenges. But keeping minds focused on our goals and learning from failure will ultimately help us achieve success.

References

1. Moris DN, Linos D. Music meets surgery: two sides to the art of "healing". Surg Endosc. 2013;27(3):719–23.
2. Louie PK, et al. Reaching for peak performance during surgical training: the value in assessment tools and critical performance measures. JAAOS – J Am Acad Orthop Surg. 2020;28(17):e744–51.
3. Moulton CA, et al. Teaching surgical skills: what kind of practice makes perfect?: a randomized, controlled trial. Ann Surg. 2006;244(3):400–9.
4. Bohan M, Pharmer JA, Stokes AF. When does imagery practice enhance performance on a motor task? Percept Mot Skills. 1999;88(2):651–8.
5. Verrier ED. The elite athlete, the master surgeon. J Am Coll Surg. 2017;224(3):225–35.

4 Setting and Achieving Goals

Vijay Yanamadala and Brandon Weiss

What Is a Goal?

It is important to understand what a goal is before discussing how to successfully set and achieve them, especially in the setting of healthcare training. A goal is a result or achievement toward which effort is directed [1]. A person can have multiple individualized goals that serve different purposes or all work together to achieve a larger goal. Goals can also be used as motivational tools or just as a way to stay organized as a person tries to work their way towards a large accomplishment. Goals can be broken up into different categories depending on their purpose (attainable and unattainable goals) and the expected length of time they are expected to take (short-term and long-term goals). Through understanding what the different types of goals are, how those goals work together and how to successfully set and accomplish them, you can learn to be more efficient as you work to achieve tasks in the future.

V. Yanamadala (✉)
Hartford Healthcare, Westport, CT, USA

Quinnipiac University Frank H. Netter School of Medicine, North Haven, CT, USA
e-mail: Vijay.Yanamadala@hhchealth.org

B. Weiss
Lake Erie College of Osteopathic Medicine, Erie, PA, USA
e-mail: bweiss08007@med.lecom.edu

© The Author(s), under exclusive license to Springer Nature Switzerland AG 2022

P. K. Louie et al. (eds.), *The Successful Health Care Professional's Guide*,
https://doi.org/10.1007/978-3-030-95950-0_4

Unattainable Versus Attainable Goals

Goals can either be classified as unattainable goals and attainable goals. Unattainable goals are generally goals that are extremely difficult to achieve with the current level of resources or knowledge that the person who sets it has at their disposal [2]. While this can sometimes be a useful motivation tool, it can often lead to the person getting "emotionally attached to a goal" making it harder to deal with possible setbacks and decreasing the chance of obtaining other goal. Generally, unobtainable goals are broad and non-specific, thus hard to map out a plan. An example of an unattainable goal would be ending all disease in the world. While it is a noble cause and could be used as a good source of motivation, it is virtually impossible for any one person to achieve this goal. Attainable goals are usually specific goals that are possible to achieve with the current resources or knowledge that a person has at their disposal [2]. While these goals can still be difficult, it is possible to make plans for how to achieve them efficiently and effectively. This type of goal can lead to a boost in morale. When the task is completed, it helps to increase confidence and could lead to the completion of other tasks. An example of an attainable goal is getting a college degree. While still an exceedingly difficult and long task to complete, this goal is very achievable with hard work and careful planning.

Short Term Goals Versus Long Term Goals

Goals can also be divided into either Short-Term or Long-Term. A short-term goal is a goal that can be completed in a relatively short amount of time [3]. This can be something like getting a high grade on your test next week or completing an important task at your job on any given day. This type of goal can help you to think about what you can do right now. Short term goals generally have fewer steps to completing them and while completing one may seem small overall, they can have a snowball effect that leads to the completion of bigger goals in the future.

Long-term goals are goals that take many steps to complete and are usually representative of what is desired to be completed in the future [4]. These goals cannot be completed rapidly and require a fair amount of planning. Examples of this can be getting a college degree or getting your dream job in a desired field. Often these goals can consist of many shorter goals that may be necessary in order to efficiently achieve the long-term goal. These shorter goals enveloped in a long-term goal are called objectives. Setting objectives creates a structure of goals that makes the overall goal seem more obtainable and commonly leads to a higher level of success [5].

Creating objectives (also known as sub-goals) can often supply positive reinforcement, leading to greater levels of motivation for the overarching long-term goal which can be attributed to greater chance of success. Examples of objectives can be passing a particular class, getting high marks on a rotation, or even the completion of the healthcare-related degree. While objectives can lead to increase motivation, it is important to be careful of goal distraction. Goal distraction is when a person loses motivation for the long-term task due to a high sense of accomplishment from completing the sub-goals that they have set for themselves [5]. Thus, it is important to always keep a focus on the long-term goal as you move through your objectives, as to not fall victim to goal distraction.

Setting Goals Effectively

Now that we have discussed what a goal is and the different types of goals that there are, it is important to understand how to set a goal that can be successfully achieved. The setting of a goal can be one of the most important steps. A goal that is unachievable can lead to a person quitting before reaching their goal, while one that is too easy may lead to goal distraction from a false sense of accomplishment and prevent a person from moving forward to a larger goal. Given the arduous path of various healthcare training pathways, understanding goal setting is crucial. Thus, a "good" goal is usually one that requires significant motivation to complete it, yet not so hard that it is considered impossible with the current resources and knowledge that the person has.

One of the best ways to ensure that you are setting a strong goal is by following the S.M.A.R.T model [6–8]. This model describes specific characteristics that a goal should have in order to be effective and efficient. The acronym stands for specific, measurable, achievable, realistic/relevant and time-bound. Next, we will dive further into each of the areas of S.M.A.R.T and discuss why they are important to setting a successful goal.

Specific This component of goal setting is exactly what it sounds like. It is shown that people tend to work harder and more efficiently to achieve a goal that has well defined objectives and a known outcome [6]. Setting a broad goal can lead to frustration and decrease the speed at which a person is able to complete the goal. A specific goal should be able to answer questions such as 'What objectives need to be accomplished?' and 'what steps must be taken to achieve these objectives?' [8]. This will allow for a plan to be set to lead to the most efficient achievement of the goal. In terms of getting into the healthcare field, objectives for a specific goal may include: Getting into the advanced training fields, passing the board exams, and obtaining the desired job after years of training. Each of these goals are specific and help can help move closer to the ultimate goal of becoming a healthcare professional. If you look deeper into any one of these goals, you can see of how the second question applies in this case. For example, to achieve the goal of passing the board exams, a study schedule can be made that maps out a daily plan to ensure readiness for the exam.

Measurable While a specific goal is a good starting point, there needs to be a quantitative element to track. By also making sure that the goal has a quantitative component (i.e., a measurable component), it is easier to track progress and know how far away the finish line is at any given time [7, 8]. By going back to the board exam example that was previously discussed, a measurable component can be added by doing periodic practice questions or taking practice tests to see how close the practice score is to the desired score.

Achievable This simply means having the ability to achieve or accomplish the goal that is being set [6–8]. While setting unattainable goals can be used as a motivation tool in some cases, in others it can actually hinder progress as there is no satisfaction from reaching the finish-line and may distract from the completion of other goals. Goals such as ending disease or supplying healthcare to the entire world may seem great, but as discussed before, are impossible for anyone person to accomplish. Instead, setting a goal of becoming an infectious disease specialist to research and help cure various diseases is a much more specific and attainable goal and thus will allow for a more definite path to be formed and a higher likely hood of achieving the goal. Asking questions such as 'is the goal reasonably possible?' and 'Are there any barriers that may block the ability to attain the goal?' can help to assess whether a goal has this quality or not.

Realistic/relevant Setting a goal should have intent and drive. It is not effective to set a goal that is not relevant or it does not realistically fit in with other goals as there is less of a chance of it being achieved [8]. If a person's main goal is centered around entering a healthcare field, an additional goal of becoming the first person to walk on Mars may not make sense towards achieving their main goal and direct time and effort away from that main goal. Thus, it is important to identify why the goal is important and how it fits in with other goals that are trying to be achieved. Being able to find this key benefit will help to keep motivation levels high and lead to an increased chance of success in goal achievement.

Time-bound This component of goal writing can also fall under the measurable component as it can be quantitative but is so important that it was broken into its own piece of the goal setting puzzle. An infinite goal cannot be achieved. Without putting a timeline on your goal, there will be no source of motivation to complete it [6, 8]. It is important to be conscious of one's own ability to complete a task when setting these timelines [6]. A time-line that is too short can lead to immense pressure and lower quality of the overall work being done to achieve the goal. A timeline that is too long can lead to slacking off and less focus on obtaining the goal. By putting time related parameters, it allows you to stay on track within each objective of your goal.

After going through each step to determine the components of the goal, it is important to put it all together into one cohesive idea. Now that a cohesive goal has been created, a focus must be put on how to successfully navigate that goal from the initial setting through completion of the goal.

How to Achieve Goals?

Obviously, we all want to achieve the goals that we set for ourselves. It is even one of the specific components that we looked at when setting our goals. Thus, it is important to have a strong plan on how to successfully achieve the goals that are set. With every goal being unique there could be additional or unique steps that need to be taken, but every goal can be started in a similar manner.

One of the first things that should be done after setting a goal is writing it down and keeping it somewhere that is consistently visible [8]. Often goals can be skewed or forgotten if just left in memory. A past study by Dr. Gail Matthews at Dominican university in California has shown that people who write down their goal are 42% more likely to achieve their goal [9]. Thus, writing the goal down will ensure that the exact goal originally set is what is being completed. Additionally, seeing a goal more often will lead to increased levels of motivation to complete that goal.

After writing down your goal it is important to dive further into the plan [10]. answering questions such as the below, can help to create a focus plan and increase the chances of achieving the desired goal:

1. What is my realistic timeframe for completing this goal?
2. What are the major steps in completing this goal?
3. What resources will I need to complete this goal?
4. Is there anyone who can help me complete this goal?

Each of these questions will help to better clarify what is needed to complete the goal that was set, which in turn will allow for it to be accomplished more efficiently. Identifying the resources that are needed to complete the task is especially important as without the correct resources most tasks are virtually impossible to complete. Understanding what is need from the start is a great way to ensure that you will have everything you need as you move through each step saving precious time and energy.

Another good way to ensure a successful path toward achieving a goal is to set regular check ins along the way [8]. When the goal is first set there will be a huge spike in your motivation to complete it. Over time, this motivation will slowly fall and lead to decreased performance or slower progress on the tasks related to completing the goal. It can be likened to the flow of a semester of school. Many healthcare students have large amounts of motivation to study and do well in the beginning of a school year. As the semester wages on and fatigue begins to take hold, motivation levels begin to fall. For many students, midterms serve as a check in on their progress and can jump start their motivation again allowing them to push through the rest of the year. Setting check ins along your goals serves the same purpose.

Depending on the goal, these check ins could be frequent or fairly spaced out. For a goal such as passing the board exams, weekly check ins are common to make sure that the study plan is being followed and scores are moving in the right direction. For longer term goals such as getting the job you desire, bimonthly or even monthly check-ins may be more appropriate. Later, we will discuss the role of mentors Mentors or counselors in helping to guide these check ins.

In addition to writing your goals down and doing regular check-ins to ensure that the goals stay on track, it is important to celebrate achieving each step of your goal [8]. While getting too caught up in every little success can lead to goal distraction, not celebrating any goal milestones can also have a negative impact on achieving a goal [6–8]. Celebrating successes, no matter how small, can cause a large spike in dopamine that can actually help to increase motivation and increase the likelihood of successfully completing future tasks related to the goal being worked on. Therefore, taking a moment to reflect on and enjoy the completion of an objective in a goal before moving on to the next step can be almost as important as actually completing the objective in the first place.

One more important factor that should be considered, if possible, is the order in which the tasks are performed. For some goals, the order is already set. Virtually every modern healthcare worker today has followed a similar path with some minor variations to get to their position. However, many goals can have objectives that can be done in any order and thus one must consider this when making a plan for how to tackle those steps. While many people like to do the harder tasks first, there is evidence that doing the easier tasks first may actually be the better choice [11]. Various studies have shown that completing easier tasks first can lead to an increase in motivation and a higher likelihood of completing the more difficult tasks later. On the contrary, when the harder tasks are tackled first, there is higher chance of frustration building and a deviation from completing the task or the dropping of the task completely.

Always remember that while these techniques are helpful in ensuring a goal stays on an efficient and successful path, every goal is unique and must be approached individually. Much like how different topics throughout your schooling career required slight variations of study styles to successfully complete them, each goal can have a slightly different approach to completing them. There is no one recipe to ensure that every goal is completed 100% of the time so it is important to start with a consistent approach, but also be malleable as the goal progresses further into its objectives.

Role Models and their Effect on Goals

An especially important tip to making sure you complete goals in a timely manner is to never be afraid to ask for help. Many times, there is someone out there that has been through a similar situation that you are in and are happy to help you navigate your unique goal. Many of these helpers can become lifelong aids in the form of role models or mentors.

A role model is an individual who is able to demonstrate the behaviors and responsibilities of a specific aspect of life [12]. Role models can be virtually anyone who is in a position that other aspire to be. Attending physicians often serve as role models to the residents who work under them, and residents can serve as role models to the medical students. While there are a lot of characteristics of a role model that can be found in literature, three particular themes seem to always be present in some form or another [12]. A role model:

(a) Demonstrates how to successfully preform a given task or complete a goal.
(b) Prove that a given goal is attainable (as they have already achieved it).
(c) Serve as inspirations for others who want to achieve the goal.

Through these 3 characteristics, a role model can be a powerful aid in helping someone achieve their goals. By showing that the goal is attainable, it gives a higher sense of motivation and prevents the discouragement of an impossible task. Being an inspiration can also be useful as it can help to reinforce the goal (almost like the check ins that were discussed earlier). Finally, by helping others learn to successfully achieve their goals, the role model can help others avoid or persevere through road blocks simply through their past actions.

While a person can have many role models in their life who can help them to navigate upcoming goals through their past and current actions, only a select few of these role models will become a mentor to the person. Role models can be anyone in a position that matches your goals; you do not need to have even met them. Mentors are usually wise and trusted advisors that a person has a close relationship with [13, 14]. At the center of that relationship is a teaching-learning process that is backed up by support and guidance.

An effective mentor can have large impacts on many aspects in a person's professional life. They can help with professional development, learning to network effectively and how to advance further towards achieving a goal. Through actions such as coaching, assessing and sponsoring, a mentor can help a mentee to design detailed plans to avoid major roadblocks in the process of goal achievement.

While their roles may be slightly different, both role models and mentors are extremely useful resources to help a person achieve their goals. It would be wise to always take their words or past experiences into consideration when deciding how to proceed forward on a goal. Their experience and advice can help to avoid potential barriers to completing your goals or can help to speed up the timeline for goal achievement. Thus, as stated before, do not be afraid to ask for help when you feel stuck.

How to Deal with Failure

Everyone deals with setbacks and failures in life. Dealing with failure is an important part of the goal making process. Failure does not mean an immediate abandonment of the goal, but rather that a different approach is needed to be taken. Perseverance is a vital trait to have in order to ensure that goals will be achieved in the most efficient manner possible. However, a pivot from your previous approach to a new approach should not be a random event. Research has shown that people who fail and give up and those who succeed often retried the goal the same number of times [15]. The major difference between those who were successful and those who were unsuccessful is how the person handled the pivot to the new approach.

People who move on to a new approach to the problem in a seemingly random manner with no reason for the new approach tend not to be successful. Often, they end up running into many of the same obstacles that they ran into with the previous approach and making many unnecessary changes that lead to even more issues. No matter their level of perseverance, this approach does not generally produce success in an efficient manner and can be more work in the long run [15].

Instead, it was those who chose to learn from their previous approach that tended to be successful [15]. Thus, the first step to rebound from a setback or failure is to regroup and reassess [16]. Taking the time to review what went wrong in the previous attempt to achieving a goal is useful to avoid future failures. A good example of this can be seen when applying to any graduate level healthcare programs. These programs can be hard to get into and can sometimes take multiple times of applying before the hurdle can be cleared. If after failing to get accepted, you simply reapply or randomly change things on your application you are likely to have a similar result. If instead you take the time to review your weak areas with a mentor or advisor, you will have a better idea of how to increase your chances of success in your next round of applications.

After the reason for the failure has been ascertained, the next step is to identify new paths that can be taken to avoid the previous barriers that prevented success in the original plan [15, 16]. This can be an exceedingly difficult task as many people tend to have a lot of frustration which makes it hard to move on from the previous approach. Getting an outside prospective from a mentor or peer can help to ease some of this frustration and focus on new paths that can be taken. It is okay to identify more than one potential path. At this point it is more important to flush out all of the options that could lead to future success. This could be seen in our previous example as finding ways to address the weaknesses that are identified. If three weak areas were identified in the previous step, multiple new paths to strengthen each one of them should be created.

After all the possible paths have been identified, each path must be reviewed extensively to narrow it down to what the best option moving forward is. This is where the actual pivot occurs to the new path. For the medical school application example, if one of the weaknesses on the application is a lack of volunteer hours then that area can be strengthened by doing many small volunteer events, each for a small number of hours, or working with one organization for a large number of hours. Both of these paths can help to strengthen the application and achieve the overall goal of getting into medical school, but it is important to consider which path strengthens the application more and is better for the person. This can be one of the scariest steps after a failure or setback. The fear of picking the wrong path can lead to delays and decreases in motivation to complete the task. No matter which path is chosen, it is important to make sure that the path chosen can still be completed with the resources at hand. Even more importantly, once a path is chosen, it must be pursued fully. Walking back to a different approach when midway through a chosen path can lead to additional failures and mounting frustration.

References

1. "Goal." 1. Collins English Dictionary. 2012 online edition. 2012. www.dictionary.com/browse/goal.
2. Ruggeri A. Why we should all give up on goals already. BBC.com. BBC. 17 Nov. 2017. www.bbc.com/worklife/article/20171117-why-we-should-all-give-up-on-goals-already.
3. What is a short-term goal? MyMnCareers. Minnesota State Colleges and Universities. 2021. https://careerwise.minnstate.edu/mymncareers/english-learner/short-term-goal.html.
4. What is a long-term goal? MyMnCareers. Minnesota State Colleges and Universities. 2021. https://careerwise.minnstate.edu/mymncareers/english-learner/long-term-goal.html.
5. Huang S-C, et al. Step by step: sub-goals as a source of motivation. Organ Behav Hum Decis Process. 2017;141:1–15. https://doi.org/10.1016/j.obhdp.2017.05.001.
6. Lunenburg FC. Goal-setting theory of motivation. Int J Manag Bus Adm. 2011;15(1):1–6. https://static1.squarespace.com/static/5b0b8f55365f02045e1ecaa5/t/5b14d215758d46f9851858d1/1528091160453/Lunenburg%2C+Fred+C.+GoalSetting+Theoryof+Motivation+IJMBA+V15+N1+2011.pdf.
7. Ogbeiwi O. Why written objectives need to be really SMART. Br J Healthc Manag. 2017;23:336. https://doi.org/10.12968/bjhc.2017.23.7.324.
8. Boogaard K. How to write SMART goals. Work Life, Atlassian. 15 Nov. 2020. www.atlassian.com/blog/productivity/how-to-write-smart-goals.
9. Gardner S, Albee D. Study focuses on strategies for achieving goals, resolutions. Press Releases. 266. 2015. https://scholar.dominican.edu/news-releases/266.
10. The S.A.M. guide to goal setting. CeDAR. UCHealth. 2021. www.cedarcolorado.org/articles/peer-support/the-s-a-m-guide-to-goal-setting/.
11. Jin L, Xu Q, Zhang Y. Climbing the wrong ladder: the mismatch between consumers' preference for subgoal sequences and actual goal performance. J Mark Res. 2015;52:628. https://doi.org/10.1509/jmr.13.0014.
12. Morgenroth T, Ryan MK, Peters K. The motivational theory of role modeling: how role models influence role aspirants' goals. Rev Gen Psychol. 2015;19:483. https://doi.org/10.1037/gpr0000059.
13. Thorndyke LE, Gusic ME, Milner RJ. Functional mentoring: a practical approach with multilevel outcomes. J Contin Educ Health Prof. 2008;28:164. https://doi.org/10.1002/chp.178.
14. Ratnapalan S. Mentoring in medicine. Can Fam Physician. 2010;56(2):198.
15. Yin Y, et al. Quantifying the dynamics of failure across science, startups and security. Nature. 2019;575(7781):190–4. Web.
16. Marks ML, et al. Rebounding from career setbacks. Harvard Business Review. Harvard Business School. Oct. 2014. hbr.org/2014/10/rebounding-from-career-setbacks.

Career Planning

5

Bryan T. Kelly and Noareen Zaheer Ahmed

Many industries and careers outside of the healthcare space can be uniquely identified by defined by a structured, defined pathway to senior leadership roles. Career planning, then, becomes closely tied to determining how and when select milestones can be met and fulfilled. Although this book focuses broadly on healthcare trainees in general, this chapter shines the spotlight more heavily on physician, and more specifically, surgeons. However, we feel as though our experiences and information are widely generalizable across multiple healthcare fields, and will work to present it as such.

For physicians, career planning begins as early as medical school, as the student is exposed to a comprehensive array of medical specialties, one of which will define their career trajectory. The Association of American Medical Colleges outlines a four-phase career planning process for medical students grounded in the theory of person-environment fit (previously Parsons' trait and factor theory). The four phases include: (1) Understand Yourself; (2) Explore Options; (3) Choose Your Specialty; (4) Prepare for Residency. In the first phase, a variety of self assessment tools can be used to better understand their interests, values, skills, and personality. Assessment tools such as: Medical Specialty Preference Inventory (MSPI); Physician Values in Practice Scale (PVIPS); and Physician Skills Inventory (PSI), can be used by students to some of these questions. In order to make the most informed decision about ones future career, a complete exploration of specialty options and practice settings must be performed to understand critical aspects including residency program requirements, competitiveness, workforce, compensation and the impact on work-life balance. Choosing a specialty is perhaps the most important decision that junior doctors need to make – and often times have to make the decision with a limited understanding of the implications of this choice. Getting as much information as possible about different specialties is critical, to make sure that the decision will be

B. T. Kelly · N. Z. Ahmed (✉)
Office of Medical Leadership, Hospital for Special Surgery, New York, NY, USA
e-mail: kellyb@hss.edu; ahmedn@hss.edu

© The Author(s), under exclusive license to Springer Nature Switzerland AG 2022

P. K. Louie et al. (eds.), *The Successful Health Care Professional's Guide*,
https://doi.org/10.1007/978-3-030-95950-0_5

compatible with their educational and career goals. Once the decision is made, preparation for residency is critical to make sure that the junior doctor is as prepared as possible to be positioned for a successful residency experience, which will likely provide the foundation for career potential and trajectory going forward [1].[1]

This Four-Phase Career Planning Process is only the first of many decisions that will define ones future in medicine. Surgical specialties have unique challenges, as the training requires the ability to balance patient care, knowledge procurement and mastery, technical skill acquisition in the operating room, and the development of research, academic and innovation skills. As a surgeon, there are key professional milestones to consider across various domains beyond clinical and surgical performance. This can include academics, research, leadership development, innovation and more. Often, these milestones can be concurrent, e.g., a promotion to associate professorship and a promotion to a clinical leadership role, or one may precede the other. General parameters exist, but more often than not, it is up to the individual physician, and in this case, surgeon, to set these goals for him/herself.

Such is the traditional basis for career planning: what should one aim to do, when should it be completed, and how does one reach the next step? Historically, defining these "checkpoints" and "milestones" were ways in which surgeons would "career plan". Traditional career planning more often than not relied on a "one size fits all" model. Milestones were, and in some cases are still, often anchored to volume--the number of years in practice, patient volume, publications, accolades, and more. Clearly defined checkpoints drove the way in which many advanced professionally.

However, in this day and age, the environment within and outside of the healthcare industry is shifting rapidly. As surgeons, our priorities, too, are shifting as a product of this turbulent environment. Market pressures, industry forces and shifts, new entrants, environmental factors, and a shift away from "traditional", and in some cases archaic, practices, are and will continue to impact the way in which surgeons plan their careers and approach career development more wholly.

Amidst a shape-shifting, and now "post-pandemic" reality, it is becoming increasingly important to have an adaptable, agile approach to career planning. That means, know where to go and the vision to be fulfilled—but have flexibility in the way in which that advancement is achieved, that milestone is fulfilled, and that goal is completed. The development of a comprehensive Individual Development Plan (IDP) can help organize the thought process of the surgeon as they start the early stages of their careers (Appendix 1).

Many surgeon leaders across the country follow and embrace "best-in-class" professional habits. These leading practices, skills and framework(s) can facilitate the way in which operative and non-operative physicians engage in their individual career planning process throughout the span of their professional and medical careers.

These guiding principles, informed by leading practices, are outlined in the following section.

[1] https://www.aamc.org/cim/general/four-phase-career-planning-process

Career Planning Best Practices

Guiding Principle 1: Seek Feedback Through Mentorship

Corporate careers, such as banking, finance, and consulting, are recognized for a culture of ongoing feedback. Performance metrics, although objective, are paired with subjective, qualitative feedback—often systematically integrated into the performance management and development structure of any given organization.

Throughout surgical training--from medical school, to residency, fellowships and beyond--feedback, when shared, is methodical and often tied to clinical performance. This type of traditional feedback is critical. Clinical performance and accomplishments are integral factors that contribute to long, successful careers in healthcare.

Being a strong surgeon, with leading outcomes and metrics, allows a surgeon to create a sound foundation upon which he or she can not only plan for future practice development, but also layer in other domains that can "diversify" a surgeon's toolkit and areas of professional focus—academics, research, leadership, innovation, communication, citizenship to a given group or organization and more.

As surgeons now diversify their professional interests, whether it be by taking on administrative/ leadership roles, developing industry relationships with new entrants and players in the care delivery space, or simply evolving their scope, *broader* feedback and advice is critical.

Historically, surgeons are all too familiar with high-pressure, competitive environments. Amidst this setting especially, seeking opportunities to advance professionally, across clinical and non-clinical skillsets, is a key enabler for future success. Focusing on constructive, actionable feedback can ultimately foster a culture of collective collaboration, teamwork and betterment for the team, not only the individual. A culture where each individual is striving to better his or her trade, brand and value to the broader team is one of excellence.

Often, a means to seek feedback across the formative years of a surgeon's career is through formal or informal mentorship. Mentorship by nature is an individualized relationship—this is to say, mentorship means something different to everyone, especially in surgery. Most commonly, a mentor serves as a senior or informed individual who can guide a trainee, a junior staff or truly anyone who seeks to develop in his or her career, in personal, educational, professional and clinical matters.

As a surgeon plans a career, long-term mentors can provide guidance stemming from personal/ professional experience, while also providing constructive and tailored feedback longitudinally across a surgeon's career. Surgical mentorship, which does not take a one-size-fits-all approach, can range from technical mentorship, to financial mentorship, to industry mentorship and many more sub-specializations. Through strong mentors comes clear pathways for continued feedback, guidance and advice.

Guiding Principle 2: Remain Agile

Providers, operative and non-operative alike are often guided by a larger mission—upholding the Hippocratic Oath, fulfilling the mission of a given healthcare organization or practice, or simply—caring for patients in the safest, most effective way possible.

Anchoring career development to tactical goals may have been enough in the era preceding today; this model may be archaic in a time where now the only constant seems to be change. Accelerated change, at that.

There is merit and value in planning, but often—those who can easily navigate turbulence amidst the immediate and external environment are those who not only understand where they are going, but also appreciate that there needs to be flexibility in how they can get there.

This is the premise of agility and adaptability. By constantly revisiting milestones, goals and professional targets, surgeons can further enable their success. Adaptability may seems counterintuitive to the precision and structure of the art that is surgery. However, the ability to refresh, recalibrate and adjust as conditions evolve is a means to position oneself for continued success. This is because it ensures that the needs of each situation are appropriately met.

The importance of adaptability and agility was as evident as ever with the COVID-19 pandemic. Many surgeons nation-wide, and even globally, were met with professional challenges that required a complete recalibration in process and day-to-day. These daily adaptations, through changing workflows, protocols, processes, safety practices, clinical care delivery and more, relied heavily on the ability to react to the immediate environment, all while being grounded in the highest-level goal of providing care to those who needed it most.

The COVID-19 pandemic, the impact it had during the peak, and the impact it left in its wake, magnified the importance of flexibility, and the willingness to embrace flexibility, amidst an ongoing journey of professional development.

Guiding Principle 3: Focus on Contribution & Professional Fulfillment, Not Individual Accomplishments

The training to become a surgeon is powerfully shaped—competitive forces and pressures are often synonymous with unique specialties, deadlines, and academic milestones. Success is, then, often measured in terms of individual goals—from undergraduate coursework through medical school and beyond.

This notion of "acquisition", that is—working towards acquiring individual accolades, recognition and milestones, has been referred to as the "first mountain" [2]. Truly progressive, proactive career planning should include an openness and willingness to explore the "second peak," which is the concept of contribution. This shift is rooted in committing to a concept, vision or mission that is bigger than oneself.

At its very core, this concept is about making a commitment without expecting a return. Anchoring to that concept enables surgeons to embark on a path of professional fulfillment, professional development and an everlasting focus to redefine excellence and what it means to be "best-in-class."

Planning a career that is fueled by genuine energy, motivation and commitment to simply contributing to something bigger than oneself, in many cases this can be committing to a mission or vision, is a means by which one can achieve professional fulfillment in his or her work [2]. Doing so enables surgeons at any stage in their careers to not be driven by individual accolades, but rather will enable opportunities to seek true competitive advantage—that is, reaching and navigating the second peak of contribution.

Guiding Principle 4: Develop Leadership Skills

As an individual works through both the act of career planning and also making progress across career-goals, it is common to seek or begin to embrace leadership opportunities. To be a leader may have different formal implications, but even through the early stages of a career—there is space for leadership development.

For surgeons navigating increasingly complex health care institutions, leadership, management and business skills become as critically important as medical expertise. Strategic opportunities for professional growth can empower junior surgeons to emerge as leaders. Leadership competencies may vary across organizations and surgical specialties, but at the core—a strong surgeon leader excels across: clinical performance, people management, crisis management, communication, decision-making, data literacy, promoting a stronger team, organizational citizenship, quality, safety & improvement and overall business/ operations acumen.

Although strong clinical expertise is essential to a successful career, integrating broader leadership skills and tools is essential to being a successful, impactful and meaningful leader.

Key Takeaways

Through thoughtful, comprehensive and individualized career planning built on a foundation of strong clinical expertise, feedback, advice, agility, fulfillment and leadership skill development, surgeons can position themselves for continued success.

Career planning can be challenging, especially with continued environmental uncertainty, but the shared guiding principles can be the constant thread through ongoing change. These principles, practices and recommendations can be used as a guide to help a surgeon begin, progress or advance a surgical career (and certainly any healthcare-related career) that maximizes potential, growth and development.

Appendix 1: Individual Development Plan (Academy of Medical Educators [3])

Clearly outlining short- and long-term career goals is a necessary initial step in achieving them. An Individual Development Plan (IDP) is a document enumerating professional goals and projecting time frames in which to accomplish them. It is a formal 'to do' list to help guide your efforts in multiple areas of your career.

Self-assessment of Professional Skills, Interests and Values

It is necessary to view your career aspirations in the context of various pillars that guide professional development, such as what are your professional interests and values, and what are the skills you have and need to acquire. Completing a self-assessment survey addressing these pillars can help you identify the items to include in your IDP. One such survey is the MyIDP (http://myidp.sciencecareers.org/) which asks you to rate your proficiency and interests in multiple professional areas including technical skills, ability to communicate, managerial skills, and promotion goals.

Defining What You Want to Achieve

As a first step, think about what you want to achieve during your career. What are your overall professional aspirations? How do you want to make a difference in your field?

Consider Your Current Professional Strengths

Reflect on your professional strengths. Think of your positive attributes, like your technical skills, knowledge base, inter-personal skills, and other aspects of your professional behavior that are strengthens. In other words, what do you do well?

Consider Your Current Professional Weaknesses

Now reflect on your professional weaknesses. This includes what you need to improve upon, what could you do better? Think of gaps in your knowledge, skills you need to acquire, and resources and connections you need to seek.

Consider What Opportunities Are Available

Consider what opportunities for growth exist in your field. What are gaps in knowledge and expertise that will become increasing important in your field? Where will future attention and resources be focused? Which of these areas are you well suited to pursue? Also consider what tangible opportunities for advancement exist in your environment, such as openings in your department, institution or national organization.

Consider Potential Threats to Your Plans

It is important to acknowledge what barriers may exist that make achieving your goals harder. These are things that you may not be able to influence, such as changes in funding or re-organization of your department. Your plans need to take into account these external challenges so that you can modify and potentially re-channel some of your goals.

©Hospital for Special Surgery 2017–2019

Generate Items for the IDP: Address Four Attributes

Select several major career aspirations. Think of each one in terms of these four attributes:

what is the ***goal*** (what is the objective); what will you do to accomplish the goal (what ***actions*** will you need to do); what will be the ***outcome*** (what will be the tangible result); and.

when will the goal be accomplished (what is the ***target date*** for completion).

Think of what strengths you have and what weaknesses you need to address to fulfill each aspiration. Also consider how external forces may offer opportunities or present barriers for each aspiration.

In order to turn these aspirations into items for your IDP, you must make them actionable – i.e. progress from describing them (in terms of nouns) to executing them (in terms of verbs). One way to do this is by using the S.M.A.R.T. criteria whereby you express each aspiration/item so that it is:

S Specific (precise, focused, one objective)
M Measurable (clear evidence that achieved)
A Attainable (realistic)
R Relevant (consequential, it matters to people in the field)
T Time allotted is appropriate for what needs to be achieved

Jot down important items according to these criteria. Express each item in terms of a goal, actions to achieve the goal, a desired outcome, and a target date for completion.

©Hospital for Special Surgery 2017–2019

Sample IDP Here are samples of generic items that may be applicable to your current professional role. Each item has a *goal*, *actions* to achieve the goal, a desired *outcome*, and a *target date* for completion. A space also is allocated to record progress.

GOAL	ACTION	OUTCOME	TARGET DATE
Update CV	*Assemble presentations, abstracts, manuscripts with citations/dates, obtain and follow most recent CV format*	*Completed current CV*	*November 1*
	PROGRESS		
Increase OR volume by 20%	*Contact 10 colleagues in other fields and meet with senior orthopedic surgeons for referrals*	*Increased OR volume by 20%*	*April 30*
	PROGRESS		
Get promoted to associate level	*Speak to chair of promotions committee; discuss with division chief; assemble list of references; complete application*	*Application submitted*	*March 1* *March 15* *April 15*
	PROGRESS		
Submit manuscript for project A	*Clean data, analyze data, write entire manuscript,have all co-authors sign off*	*Submitted to the XYZ Journal*	*June 1*
	PROGRESS		
Expand national and international reputation	*Offer to present at Grand Rounds and be visiting professor (x4)* *Get nominated and appointed to Planning Committee of national society.*	*Presented at other institutions* *Appointed to Committee*	*November 15* *June 1*
	PROGRESS		

©Hospital for Special Surgery 2017–2019

Assemble Your IDP

Select several current career aspirations and enter them in the template. Make your goals and actions specific, your outcomes measurable, and your target dates realistic. Use the progress area to document your efforts and record your achievements along the way. Review your competed IDP with your mentor and modify if necessary. Keep this IDP in a visible place to help keep you on track.

GOAL	ACTION	OUTCOME	TARGET DATE
PROGRESS			
PROGRESS			
PROGRESS			
PROGRESS			

References

1. Four-phase career planning process [Internet]. Aamc.org. [cited 2021 Jun 15]. Available from: https://www.aamc.org/cim/general/four-phase-career-planning-process.
2. Brooks D. Opinion. The New York times [Internet]. 2019. [cited 2021 Jun 15]; Available from: https://www.nytimes.com/2019/04/06/opinion/sunday/moral-revolution-david-brooks.html.
3. Hospital for Special Surgery. Individual development plan- academy of medical educators. 2017–2019.

6 Resilience: How to Avoid Burnout, Provide Exceptional Care, and Successfully Integrate Work and Life

Barbara Waxman

Preparing for a healthcare career is not easy. The required education and training can take years and be grueling, with a steep cost – both financially and in terms of lifestyle sacrifices. Most emerging healthcare professionals understand this and willingly make short-term sacrifices for a career they anticipate will be personally, professionally, and financially rewarding. They expect intense training; what they are less likely to expect or receive is instruction and guidance on how to maximize that training to create a satisfying and sustainable career and lifestyle, avoid burnout and even reach peak performance in their given field.

Stanford Medicine's WellMD & WellPhD Center is involved in research dedicated to advancing well-being for doctors and biomedical professionals, based on the growing understanding that physician well-being and providing exceptional patient care are inextricably linked [1]. The Center identifies three inter-related factors necessary for experiencing fulfillment in the practice of medicine:

1. practice efficiency utilizing manageable administrative burdens that do not impede meaningful patient care;
2. an institutional culture of wellness with workplace wellness offerings and relationship-centered practices;
3. personal resilience [1].

This chapter focuses on the third factor—personal resilience. A growing body of research, including Stanford's, substantiates what is intuitive: Healthy, resilient healthcare providers, have greater levels of alertness, energy, and self-awareness and are better equipped to listen well, diagnose astutely, and treat compassionately [2]. In short, delivering effectual, patient-centered care means first taking care of oneself. Beyond education, this chapter provides the missing piece: an assessment

B. Waxman (✉)
Odyssey Group Coaching LLC, San Francisco, CA, USA
e-mail: Barbara@barbarawaxman.com

© The Author(s), under exclusive license to Springer Nature Switzerland AG 2022

P. K. Louie et al. (eds.), *The Successful Health Care Professional's Guide*,
https://doi.org/10.1007/978-3-030-95950-0_6

tool and guidance to create a personalized plan to build resilience, avoid burnout, and ultimately, achieve sustainable peak performance.

The Pain Point: Burnout

Burnout is real. Despite extraordinary advancements in medical science throughout the modern era, the actual practice of the art of medicine has become laden with bureaucratic hurdles. Burdensome insurance documentation and productivity demands, coupled with a decline in support and reimbursement, significantly contribute to nurses, physicians, and other healthcare providers in the United States reporting a higher likelihood of burnout than those working in fields with more minor bureaucratic hurdles [3]. Numerous surveys and studies report an alarming epidemic of burnout among American healthcare professionals, with nearly 50% reporting burnout symptoms [4]. And this was before the impacts of the COVID-19 pandemic, which according to a *Medical Economics* survey, resulted in 65% of front-line care providers reporting increased fatigue, stress, and safety concerns [5]. The fact that a global crisis can up-end so much further highlights the critical imperative to cultivate and maintain a high level of personal resilience.

As if the personal toll on healthcare professionals were not enough, the stresses experienced by clinicians and even trainees impact the practice of care itself. Put simply, a burned-out healthcare provider is not able to provide optimal care. Burnout can lead to increased treatment errors, increased risk of malpractice, and decreased satisfaction for healthcare professionals and their patients [6]. If the fundamental oath is to "do no harm," burnout undermines the very foundation of health care and threatens public health.

Resilience, Mindset, and Energy

When the goal is to prevent burnout, it helps to think of the term "burnout" literally. According to Merriam Webster, burning fuel is "to consume fuel," and fuel, as we know, is an energy source [7]. Thus, a burned-out care provider is someone depleted of energy. However, rarely does this happen in one significant flare-up or dramatic combustion; more often than not, burnout for health professionals is a slow, gradual process, an insidious smoldering that can be hard to recognize [8].

It is also important to remember and honor the reasons for entering this field in the first place. Most healthcare professionals are drawn to this path by a desire to help people. For them, it is a calling rather than a job, which can be a double-edged sword when this drive to care for others overshadows personal well-being. In general, being of service to others is energy-affirming and rewarding [9, 10]. The strong sense of purpose connected to that service can compensate for many of the expected hurdles experienced on the path, notably, long workdays, lost hours of sleep, and relational strains.

Burnout stems less from the hard work and long hours of patient care than from the double-binds of moral injury, the prevalence of "acts that transgress deeply held moral beliefs and expectations", forcing healthcare professionals into an impossible balancing act between the demands of patient care and the systemic constraints of providing that care. Administrators and legislators must address the overarching and systemic roots of burnout, namely moral injury [11]. Still, there is a substantial opportunity at a personal level for healthcare professionals to cultivate personal resilience by understanding how to use energy and activating a transformative mindset, behaviors, and habits to foster sustained peak performance, even in the face of challenges [12].

Resilience

There is growing research and interest in the concept of resilience, the capacity for humans to prevail in the face of hardships or factors out of one's control. Building resilience is a key factor in promoting health and well-being. Resilience is not merely the avoidance of stress. It is the ability to bounce back from stressors and maintain a sense of physical, emotional, cognitive, and spiritual equanimity. Becoming resilient is a practice that anyone can benefit from, which is essential for those entering the healthcare field. While genetics play a role, the capacity to become resilient is not reserved for the few and is not a singular accomplishment but is a result of ongoing practice.

Resilient healthcare professionals can better adapt to rapidly changing situations and incoming demands while maintaining the ability to listen carefully, integrate new information, find solutions, and act on them [12]. It is a given that there will be stressors when working in a highly demanding and dynamic field when life and death may be on the line. Thus, understanding resilience and the practices necessary to enhance it is essential for health care trainees. At the end of this chapter, the assessment tool and recommended practices serve as a resource and lay out a plan for becoming more resilient.

Mindset

In her seminal book Mindset, psychologist Carol Dweck describes how decades of research has shown that "...the view you adopt for yourself profoundly affects the way you lead your life. It can determine whether you become the person you want to be and whether you accomplish the things you value" [13]. This mental perspective is called mindset, and it forms the basis of success in every area of one's life. It is fair to assume that this chapter's readers already grasp the importance of certain aspects of mindset, likely, determination and discipline. However, what Dweck explores is a deeper understanding of how our minds and bodies are wholly interconnected and how mindset and perception impact our reality.

Dweck distinguishes between two types of mindsets: fixed and growth [13]. People with a fixed mindset perceive traits and abilities as predetermined, or as Popeye says, "I yam what I yam" [14]. Those with a fixed mindset often see failure as being due to limited abilities and espouses criticism as a personal attack [15]. However, a growth mindset views traits, abilities, and intelligence as dynamic capacities that can grow with nurturing and structured investment [15]. An individual with a growth mindset often accepts criticism as constructive feedback and embraces failure as an opportunity for growth [16]. Not surprisingly, personal resilience in healthcare providers is tied to a growth mindset [17, 18].

The topic of mindset has gained attention as researchers in positive psychology continue to expand the understanding of how the brain and body are interconnected and how a positive mindset strongly influences health and well-being. Cultivating a positive mindset has been associated with longer life, enhanced well-being, and improved health [19, 20]. It should come as no surprise, one of Harvard University's most popular courses in its history was Psychology 1504: Positive Psychology.

However, nurturing a healthy inner life is only part of the equation. Cultivating a peer support network is also essential, a form of emotional first aid, if you will. According to experts from Peers for Progress, a program of the American Academy of Family Physicians, peer support is a vital humanizing force in healthcare, a way to "harness interpersonal relations to activate intrapersonal change" [21]. As researcher Harry Harlow discovered in his famous monkey study of the 1950s, "contact comfort" and the relationships that provide it are valuable, and even vital, in and of themselves [22]. Peer support can provide both understanding and accountability, which, as noted at the end of this chapter, is a crucial tactic for building resilience.

Energy

A professional's most valuable currency is not money or even time. It is understanding how to expend the energy one has in the time available. Contrary to popular belief, the key to excelling in professional training is not merely acing tests and mastering material, but learning how to manage energy for sustainable peak performance. The problem is that it is more common to view energy as an endless resource and treat ourselves and others like human *doings* rather than human *beings*. To understand how to activate the kind of renewal that results in enhanced resilience it is instructive to think about energy as three distinct types: personal energy, interpersonal energy and universal energy.

Personal energy is like an internal reservoir that requires daily replenishment as levels become depleted. The problem is that most people treat personal energy as if it has the vast reserves of the ocean and draw it down to dangerously low levels, and at times, ultimately to complete depletion resulting in burnout. Personal energy cannot be summoned at will but must be cultivated and replenished. One way to create a sustainable reservoir of personal energy rests on a foundation of setting micro-ambitious S.M.A.R.T. goals (highlighted later in the activation steps at the end of this chapter). For example, research estimates, of the 50% of people who set New Year's Resolutions, nearly 90% are abandoned within a month [23]. Too often this is a result of aspirations that are too big, too ocean-like, rather than a more specific, achievable, reservoir-filling goals.

Interpersonal energy is derived from relationships with others and is gained or lost due to the quality of those interactions. If personal energy is a reservoir, interpersonal energy is more like an emotional bank account. Some relationships effectively deposit energy into that account, while others withdraw energy. When used constructively, interpersonal energy can bolster a sense of equanimity, connection, and resilience, while unhealthy interpersonal relationships directly impact health [24, 37].

Universal energy is free, accessible, and available to be drawn from at will, even when time and resources are scarce. It takes many forms, both natural and man-made. When activated, universal energy can heighten awareness, focus, and emotional equanimity while also decreasing one's stress response. Cultivating universal energy is a highly personal and intentional practice. Ways to tap into it include listening to music, close observation of works of art, or even improvisational activities [25]. Cultivating mindfulness through the use of breath and being in nature, along with a gratitude practice, are also ways in which universal energy can lead to higher levels of well-being [26–28].

Recognizing the difference and knowing how and when to integrate each of the three types of energy is essential. To build personal resilience, cultivating and integrating them requires daily practice, self and situational awareness, and a conscious effort. For example, a morning *personal energy* ritual as small as making coffee, a moment of reflection to ensure at least some social connections yield a profit in the *interpersonal energy* bank account and identifying small renewal moments drawn from *universal energy* yield enhanced wellness and productivity.

Choosing the Right Yardstick: Work-Life Integration

Nurturing a growth mindset, becoming resilient, and managing energy are central elements for achieving what is popularly called "work-life balance." However, aspiring towards "balance" is the wrong yardstick or, at minimum, not a helpful one [29]. The myth of work-life balance can be a set-up for failure, especially in a field more closely linked to one's identity and passion, than a vocation. Some days, rotations and cases will inevitably require more, both physically and emotionally, than others. Those times will, by necessity, feel out of balance. If the yardstick is to find balance, one will often fall short with a sense of failure that only adds to the potential for burnout [30–32]. The more realistic yardstick is to strive for work-life integration [35].

Using the concepts and resources discussed above, integrating the demands of work with a healthy personal life is achievable. Integration is dynamic and fluid, the opposite of all-or-nothing. It does not assume a binary opposition or tug-of-war between work and personal life but builds upon synergies between the two [33]. Healthcare is a field rich with meaningful relationships, intellectual growth, and personal satisfaction, often outweighing the demands. Work-life integration views these as complementary rather than conflicting with personal life goals such as family, community relationships, and personal health [34, 35]. Aiming for integration rather than balance leads to a win-win and, ideally, a decreased sense of burnout and dissatisfaction. Nevertheless, as with resilience and mindset, cultivating work-life integration to achieve peak performance takes awareness, effort, and ongoing practice.

Just as athletes, musicians, and other high performers know, success rests upon a structured and disciplined personal investment to achieve consistent and optimal results. In healthcare, the same holds. It is not enough to aim for integration; one must actively work toward it. Developing the strategies, behaviors, and habits that support resilience and increase a sense of thriving is the fine-tuning that enables emerging healthcare providers to avoid burnout, decrease emotional exhaustion, and experience a higher sense of personal accomplishment.

Assess and Understand Your Energy Baseline: The Five to Thrive Quiz©

As healthcare providers know, the first step in treatment is a thorough assessment, followed by a diagnosis, and the development of a treatment plan. As such, each individual has their baseline or starting point for treatment. In this case, the Five to Thrive Quiz provides that baseline assessment. The so-called treatment plan is a step-by-step series of intentional behavior shifts that will yield specific results. For some, the planning goal may be about reaching a level of peak performance. The starting point for others may be about avoiding burnout. This assessment is appropriate in all cases.

The 25 evidence-based questions assess the "energy building blocks," the necessary elements that ancient traditions and modern research agree, bolster personal resilience and decrease stress, resulting in enhanced wellness and enabling peak performance.

For each statement, determine the best measure of your current state and record the points. Tally the totals for each section.

How true is each statement regarding your current energy state?

0	1	2	3	4
Never	Rarely	Sometimes	Mostly	Always

Exercise & Nutrition	
I exercise 4-5x per week, balancing cardio, strength, and outdoor physical activity.	
I maintain a healthy body weight.	
I actively monitor my alcohol and sugar intake.	
I eat mostly non processed foods and more dark leafy greens than meat.	
I understand, based on my age and weight, my daily fluid intake to stay hydrated.	
Exercise & Nutrition Total:	

Rest & Renewal	
I get 7-8 hours of high-quality sleep at least 5x a week.	
I have the right number of people in my social circles who I can rely on for support and engage in some level of social interaction almost daily.	
I understand that stress is a part of life and have tools to help increase my tolerance for ambiguity and uncertainty.	
I actively monitor my screen time and technology use.	
I know how to renew my energy in small increments when I want to increase my alertness, creativity, and emotional resilience.	
Rest & Renewal Total:	

Focus & Growth

I employ mindfulness strategies like meditation that help reduce my stress levels and enhance my memory and creativity.	
I focus on things/activities that matter most to me after my workday is complete.	
I intellectually push myself by exposing myself to engage in new learning, including the exploration of new ideas and experiences.	
I take time regularly to focus on having a positive mindset rather than a negative mindset (growth versus fixed).	
I have tools that help me feel present and fully engaged in the moment.	
Focus & Growth Total:	
Joy & Passion	
I have emotionally healthy relationships at home, work, and socially.	
I engage in activities that bring me joy and a sense of fulfillment on a regular basis.	
I have a daily gratitude practice, taking time to reflect on the people and things that matter most to me.	
I regularly and frequently contribute to the causes and community needs I care about.	
Overall, my daily actions reflect my values and I allocate time and resources in ways that reflect those values.	
Joy & Passion Total:	
Time & Effort	
I prioritize my daily activities and tackle the most challenging things when I know my energy and focus is highest.	
I use technology and other tools to increase my productivity and limit my time scanning social media.	

I work in approximately 90-minute increments with a short break between activities.	
I do not multi-task to the extent I feel distracted.	
I am able to communicate my needs and say no to people.	
Time & Effort Total:	

Tally your totals to calculate your current energy state below, then circle your result.

		Current Energy State Total:		
Depleted 0–20	**Sputtering** 21–40	**Blah Zone** 41–60	**Nearly Thriving** 61–80	**Thriving** 81–100

Recommended Practices to Activate the Five Essential Elements

Now that a current energy baseline is established, the next step is to understand each of the elements and have some ideas about how to activate them successfully. The health care profession has not been immune to cultural norms that value productivity over passion, achievement over fulfillment, associate success with long hours, minimal sleep, and personal sacrifice. However, these misguided norms are a recipe for burnout and undermine a sense of engagement, focus, productivity, and connection. In contrast, nurturing resilience and a substantial energy reservoir is achievable by embracing the five essential elements of well-being.

Exercise and Nutrition

Diet and exercise are the foundational elements of a holistic approach to health, a first line of defense, and offense. In popular parlance, two adages are true: you are what you eat and use it or lose it. Research has conclusively shown that diet and exercise modifications substantially improve long-term survival and result in a portrait more nearly approaching total health [36]. Eating a plant-based diet rich in vegetables, fruits, beans and legumes, nuts/seeds, and whole grains can lower inflammation and the risk of many chronic diseases [36]. If burnout is related to fuel, then how we fuel our body and use that energy must be the primary considerations.

Recommended Practices
Eat a diet of whole, mostly plant-based foods with healthy fats.
Commit to regular exercise, optimally 150–300 minutes of moderate intensity, or 75–150 minutes of vigorous activity, along with at least two days weekly of strength training.
Actively monitor your alcohol and sugar intake.

Rest and Renewal

Skimping on sleep is frequently the default approach when one is busy or overwhelmed, and thus rest and renewal are often the most undervalued of the five elements—to our detriment. Harvard School of Medicine's Healthy Sleep project and a growing body of research confirms the many benefits of sleep, including improved learning, memory, overall health, and longevity [38–40]. Healthy sleep hygiene and mindfulness practices such as meditation, quiet walks, prayer, or yoga are central components to rest and renewal. Together, these practices can reduce stress, enhance focus, attention, and a sense of well-being [27, 39–42].

Recommended Practices
Begin and end each day with a grounding ritual, perhaps a gratitude reflection or short meditation.
Identify an effective go-to recharge method, like power naps.
Develop a strong social support system both inside and outside of work.

Focus and Growth

If energy is our most valuable currency, attention is one's most precious commodity. Focusing one's attention is more challenging given the constant barrage of incoming information from social media and the distractions from technology as a whole. As a result, most people tend to multitask, thinking they can get more done in less time. The truth is multitasking makes one less productive and less able to learn and grow one's skills [43]. Mindset and cognitive training are the bedrock of resilience [44, 45]. They can be cultivated by specific practices such as gratitude, engaging fully in one's activities, savoring pleasure, practicing mindfulness, and nurturing self-compassion [46–48]. Creativity also falls into this category as it results in a greater sense of social well-being and improved mood [49, 50].

Recommended Practices
Do not multitask, bundle complementary tasks for productivity.
Begin and end each day with a mindfulness ritual that is grounding.
Cultivate a creative pursuit.

Joy and Passion

Any high performer's most significant competitive advantage is not the sum of their accomplishments but their humanity—their meaningful relationships and emotional connection to their sense of purpose and passion. Healthcare professionals who avoid burnout maintain the ability to find joy and satisfaction in their work (despite its demands) and cultivate strong peer relationships [51]. Joy comes when actions align with values, and passion ignites energy, which helps prevent burnout. Recent research has found that people who work on something they are good at or feel passionate about report feeling greater life satisfaction and happiness [52].

Recommended Practices
Be a regular participant or contributor to the causes you care about.
Stay connected to small moments of joy that create an exponential effect.
Practice gratitude daily.

Time and Effort

Time is a non-renewable resource. To work at a level of optimal performance, one must plan to have the energy available for the associated demands [53]. It is worth repeating-- a professional's most valuable currency is not money or even time. It is understanding how to expend the energy one has in the time available and requires daily planning [53]. Those who are energetic and resilient guard their time, set boundaries, and know when to say "no" and when to jump in. They take breaks from their work approximately every 90 minutes to stretch, walk around, and re-charge for the next challenge. People who manage their time and focus their energy tend to achieve more goals and experience a better quality of life.

Recommended Practices
Set healthy boundaries and say no relentlessly.
Create a daily practice to optimize use of personal, interpersonal and universal energy.
Use technology wisely.

Activate the Five Essential Elements for Sustainable Peak Performance

With this knowledge in hand, the next step is to turn these insights into action. Developing a specific plan to hone one habit at a time will, in turn, activate an essential element of energy that will result in building resilience, strengthening capacity to avoid burnout, and ultimately achieving peak performance over the long term. It's not important where you choose to begin. For some it may be choosing the proverbial low hanging fruit; the easiest habit to create. For others, the best place will be to begin with the one change that will yield the greatest impact on energy. Making a choice you are willing to commit to is what is most important.

To activate the essential elements:

1. Choose one question to focus on from the five essential elements assessment. For example, you might choose to focus on the element of Time and Effort, choosing the question addressing multi-tasking as the best place to start.
2. Identify a habit to develop. Following the example above, a new habit may be to turn off notifications when studying or preparing to see patients.
3. Be micro-ambitious by creating one S.M.A.R.T. goal*. Using this same example, one smart goal may be to check notifications once per hour for the first 2 weeks and limit to 3 times per day by the end of 1 month.
4. Collaborate with an accountability partner. Find a partner whom you trust and don't feel judged by. Let them know exactly how you want them to hold you accountable. It may be checking in once per day, once per week—the important thing is for you to know what works for you and make a direct request.
5. Take 30 days to adopt this new habit. Taking on too many things in the short term is more draining and less sustainable then deeply embedding a new habit over a period of time.

6. Once the 30 days are complete re-assess and, if appropriate, choose a new element to improve.

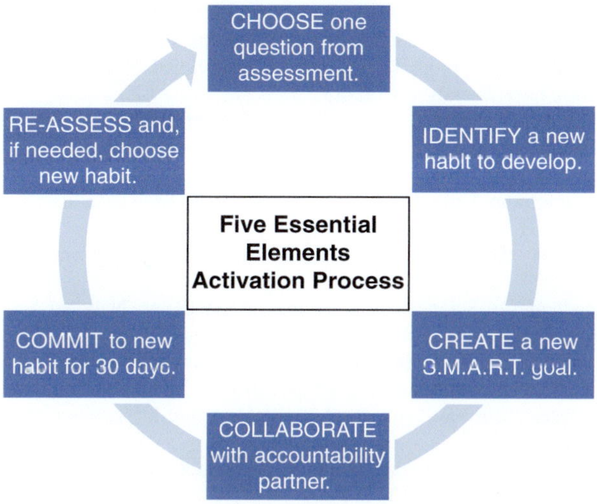

*S.M.A.R.T. goals Choosing one goal that is specific, measurable, achievable, realistic, and time-oriented, and focusing on it over the next 30 days, is a proven way to change patterns of behavior. These small goals become building blocks, not stumbling blocks, and working incrementally toward them results in feelings of accomplishment, giving one the confidence to then take on larger goals. Utilizing peer support and enlisting an accountability partner is another proven way to activate change successfully.

Conclusion

It is a given that there will be stressors when working in a highly demanding and dynamic field like healthcare. Developing and cultivating a growth mindset and recognizing that your most valuable currency is understanding how to manage your energy in the time available is foundational to avoiding burnout and reaching peak performance. Integrating the demands of work with a healthy personal life is achievable.

As Lao Tzu wisely said, “a journey of a thousand miles begins with a single step.” The more profound truth is that every step moves one either closer to or further from the desired destination and changes the experience along the way. In other words, the choices one makes day after day, step after step, define a person. On the journey to becoming a healthcare professional, the choices made, and actions taken to embrace and nurture personal well-being are some of the most important steps to take. By choosing to activate the five essential elements, one not only improves one’s sense of resilience, well-being, and work-life integration, one ultimately becomes a better care provider and has a better quality of life. In an era of an alarming burnout level, the ancient proverb, “physician heal thyself,” is more apt than ever.

References

1. The Board of Trustees of the Leland Stanford Junior University. Stanford Model of Professional Fulfillment [Internet]. Stanford Medicine: WellMD & WellPhD. [cited 2021 Apr 20]. Available from: https://wellmd.stanford.edu/about/model-external.html.
2. Shanafelt T. Physician Burnout: stop blaming the individual. NEJM Catal [Internet]. 2016:1–2. Available from: https://catalyst.nejm.org.
3. Shanafelt TD, West CP, Sinsky C, Trockel M, Tutty M, Satele DV, et al. Changes in burnout and satisfaction with work-life integration in physicians and the general US working population between 2011 and 2017. Mayo Clin. 2019;94(9):1681–94.
4. Reith TP. Burnout in United States healthcare professionals: a narrative review. Cureus. 2018;10(12):e3681.
5. Shryock T. How the COVID-19 crisis is exacerbating physician burnout. Med Econ J. 2020;97(13).
6. National Academies of Sciences, Engineering, and Medicine, National Academy of Medicine, Committee on Systems Approaches to Improve Patient Care by Supporting Clinician Well-Being. Taking action against clinician burnout: a systems approach to professional well-being. Washington, DC: National Academies Press; 2019.
7. Merriam-Webster. "Burnout" [Internet]. Available from: https://www.merriam-webster.com/dictionary/burnout.
8. De Hert S. Burnout in healthcare workers: prevalence, impact and preventative strategies. Local Reg Anesth. 2020;2020(13):171–83.
9. Hill PL, Turiano NA, Mroczek DK, Burrow AL. The value of a purposeful life: sense of purpose predicts greater income and net worth. J Res Pers. 2016;65:38–42.
10. Zika SCK. On the relation between meaning in life and psychological well-being. Br J Psychol. 1992;83:133–45.
11. Dean W, Talbot S, Dean A. Reframing clinician distress: moral injury not burnout. Fed Pract. 2019;36(9):400–2.
12. Robertson HD, Elliott AM, Burton C, Iversen L, Murchie P, Porteous T, et al. Resilience of primary healthcare professionals: a systematic review. Br J Gen Pract. 2016;66(647):e423–33.
13. Dweck CS. Mindset: The new psychology of success. New York: Random House; 2006.
14. Dweck CS. Mindsets and malleable minds: Implications for giftedness and talent. In: Subotnik RF, Robinson A, Callahan CM, Gubbins EJ, editors. Malleable minds: translating insights from psychology and neuroscience to gifted education. Storrs: University of Connecticut/National Research Center on the Gifted and Talented; 2012. p. 7–18.
15. O'Rourke E, Haimovitz K, Ballweber S, Dweck CS, Popovíc Z. Brain points: a growth mindset incentive structure boosts persistence in an educational game. In: Conference on human factors in computing systems – proceedings. Toronto: Scopus; 2014. p. 3339–48.
16. Moser JS, Schroder HS, Heeter C, Moran TP, Lee Y-H. Mind your errors: evidence for a neural mechanism linking growth mind-set to adaptive post error adjustments. Psychol Sci. 2011;22(12):1484–9.
17. Klein J, Delany C, Fischer M, Smallwood D, Trumble S. A growth mindset approach to preparing trainees for medical error. BMJ Q. 2017;26(9):771–4.
18. Stoffel JM, Cain J. Review of grit and resilience literature within health professions education. Am J Pharm Educ. 2018;82(2):6150.
19. Flanagan NM. The power of positivity. Caring Ages. 2019;20(1):3.
20. Aspinwall LG, Tedeschi RG. The value of positive psychology for health psychology: progress and pitfalls in examining the relation of positive phenomena to health. Ann Behav. 2010;39(1):4–15.
21. The American Academy of Family Physician's Foundation, UNC Gillings School for Global Public Health. Peers for progress: global support around the world. Global evidence for peer support: humanizing healthcare, September 16, 2014. Available at http://peersforprogress.

org/pfp_headline/global-evidence-for-peer-support-humanizing-health-care/. Accessed 10 Apr 2021.

22. Harlow HF, Zimmermann RR. The development of affectional responses in infant monkeys. Proc Am Philos Soc. 1958;102(5):501–9.
23. Herrick C. Why we make (and break) New Year's resolutions, and 4 tips to help you achieve your goals [Internet]. Western Connecticut Health Network Newsroom. 2020 [cited 2021 Apr 20]. Available from: https://www.westernconnecticuthealthnetwork.org/newsroom/article-listing/new-years-resolutions.
24. Simpson JA, Tran S. The needs, benefits, and perils of close relationships. In: Noller P, Feeney JA, editors. Close relationships: functions, forms and processes. Hove: Psychology Press/Taylor & Francis; 2006. p. 3–24.
25. Howley L, Gaufberg E, King B. The fundamental role of the arts and humanities in medical education. Washington, DC: AAMC; 2020.
26. Keniger LE, Gaston KJ, Irvine KN, Fuller RA. What are the benefits of interacting with nature? Int J Environ Res Public Health. 2013;10(3):913–35.
27. Hülsheger UR, Alberts HJE, Feinholdt A, Lang JWB. Benefits of mindfulness at work: the role of mindfulness in emotion regulation, emotional exhaustion, and job satisfaction. J Appl Psychol. 2012;98(2):310–25.
28. Kjellgren A, Bood SÅ, Axelsson K, Norlander T, Saatciogl F. Wellness through a comprehensive yogic breathing program – a controlled pilot trial. BMC Complementary. 2007;7:43.
29. Caproni PJ. Work/life balance: you can't get there from here. J Appl Behav. 1997;33(1):46–56.
30. Rich A, Viney R, Needleman S, Griffin A, Woolf K. "You can't be a person and a doctor": the work-life balance of doctors in training-a qualitative study. BMJ Open. 2016;6(12):e013897.
31. Shanafelt TD, Boone S, Tan L, Dyrbye LN, Sotile W, Satele D, et al. Burnout and satisfaction with work-life balance among US physicians relative to the general US population. Arch Intern. 2012;172(18):1377–85.
32. Feigon M, Block C, Breting LG, Boxley L, Dawson E, Cobia D. Work-life integration in neuropsychology: a review of the existing literature and preliminary recommendations. Clin Neuropsychol. 2017;32(2):300–27.
33. Haas School of Business. Work/life integration [Internet]. University of California. [cited 2021 Apr 20]. Available from: https://haas.berkeley.edu/human-resources/work-life-integration/.
34. Morgan J. The future of work: work life balance is becoming work life integration [Internet]. Inc. 2018 [cited 2021 Apr 20]. Available from: https://www.inc.com/jacob-morgan/work-life-balance-is-becoming-work-life-integration.html.
35. Caza BB, Ramarajan L, Reid E, Creary S. How to make room in your work life for the rest of your self [Internet]. Harvard Business Review. 2018 [cited 2021 Apr 20]. Available from: https://hbr.org/2018/05/how-to-make-room-in-your-work-life-for-the-rest-of-your-self.
36. Bodai BI, Nakata TE, Wong WT, Clark DR, Lawenda S, Tsou C, et al. Lifestyle medicine: a brief review of its dramatic impact on health and survival. Perm J. 2018;22:17–25.
37. Uchino BN, Cacioppo JT, Kiecolt-Glaser JK. The relationship between social support and physiological processes: a review with emphasis on underlying mechanisms and implications for health. Psychol Bull. 1996;119(3):488–531.
38. Division of Sleep Medicine. Why sleep matters [internet]. Harvard School of Medicine. [cited 2021 Apr 20]. Available from: http://healthysleep.med.harvard.edu/healthy/matters.
39. Luyster FS, Stroll PJ Jr, Zee PC, Walsh JK. Sleep: a health imperative. Sleep. 2012;35(6):727–34.
40. Perry GS, Patil SP, Presley-Cantrell LR. Raising awareness of sleep as a healthy behavior. Prev Chronic. 2013;10:e133.
41. Arch JJ, Landy L. Emotional benefits of mindfulness. In: Brown NKW, Creswell JD, Ryan RM, editors. Handbook of mindfulness: theory, research, and practice. London: Guilford Press; 2015. p. 208–24.
42. Schreiner I, Malcolm J. The benefits of mindfulness meditation: changes in emotional states of depression, anxiety, and stress. Behav Chang. 2008;25(3):156–68.

43. Douglas HE, Raban MZ, Walter SR, Westbrook JI. Improving our understanding of multi-tasking in healthcare: drawing together the cognitive psychology and healthcare literature. Appl Ergon. 2016;59(Part A):45–55.
44. Tabibnia G, Radecki D. Resilience training that can change the brain. Consult Psychol. 2018;70(1):59–88.
45. Joyce S, Shand F, Tighe J, Laurent SJ, Bryant RA, Harvey SB. Road to resilience: a systematic review and meta-analysis of resilience training programmes and interventions. BMJ Open. 2018;8:e017858.
46. Gogo A, Osta A, McClafferty H, Rana DT. Cultivating a way of being and doing: individual strategies for physician well-being and resilience. Curr Probl Pediatr. 2019;49(12):100663.
47. Lefebvre J-I, Montani F, Courcy F. Self-compassion and resilience at work: a practice-oriented review. Adv Dev. 2020;22(4):437–52.
48. Camgoz SM. The role of savoring in work-family conflict. Soc Behav Personal Int J. 2014;42(2):177–88.
49. Schmid T. Promoting health through creativity: for professionals in health, arts and education. Nashville: Wiley; 2008.
50. Gillam T. Creativity and mental health. In: Palgrave Studies in Creativity and Culture, editor. Creativity, wellbeing and mental health practice. Cham: Palgrave Pivot; 2018. p. 31–45.
51. Bruce SM, Conaglen HM, Conaglen JV. Burnout in physicians: a case for peer-support. Intern Med J. 2015;35(5):272–8.
52. Yukhymenko-Lescroart MA, Sharma G. The relationship between faculty members' passion for work and well-being. J Happiness. 2019;20(3):863–81.
53. Loehr J, Schwartz T. The power of full engagement: managing energy, not time, is the key to high performance and personal renewal. New York: Simon & Schuster; 2005.

Maintaining and Growing Relationships; Family, Romantic and Friends

7

Alison M. Heru

Introduction

The rigors of healthcare training are associated with significant changes in self-image that includes a newly developed sense of responsibility to others, and adaptation to a new role. These changes have been noted since the 1950's, with the recognition that these changes require much emotional strength [1]. A professional in health care learns to put the patient first, learns to deny their own comfort, and sleep, eating habits and basic self-care get put aside, in the service of others. There can be strong bonding among peers who are also going through these changes, but often these developmental steps occur out of sight and the trainee struggles alone. As more women have entered health care professions and fought and gained better maternity leave, men are now also eligible for paternity leave, reducing some of the pressure to postpone establishing a family. However, this is a small step for a family facing the real challenges of demanding schedules. Even without young children, relationships within families will be strained by the rigors of training.

It is a temptation for all trainees to want to 'veg out' at home. You want to just eat what is in the fridge, watch some mindless TV show and have a drink. The more health conscious trainees will exercise and try to shop for good meals. The most health conscious trainees will want to attend to their mental health and to the health of their relationships. But what strategies can we use to help with our relationships? There is very little in the literature that can guide trainees on how to manage their relationships, except to say that we should have supportive relationships; but what does this mean? How do you define a supportive relationship? The adage that you know it when you feel it, does little to help those in search of building or maintaining a supportive relationship. The next section examines the current literature on developing relational strengths and parses out how we understand individual

A. M. Heru (✉)
Department of Psychiatry, University of Colorado Denver, Denver, CO, USA
e-mail: alison.heru@cuanschutz.edu

© The Author(s), under exclusive license to Springer Nature Switzerland AG 2022

P. K. Louie et al. (eds.), *The Successful Health Care Professional's Guide*,
https://doi.org/10.1007/978-3-030-95950-0_7

resilience and relational resilience. Based on this understanding, we can develop programs and interventions that focus on strengthening our family relationships.

Current State of Understanding of Social Support, Individual and Relational Resilience

Family stress contributes to trainee burnout, and trainee burnout contributes to family stress; a reciprocal and downward spiraling relationship between family stress and burnout. Burnout is common among trainees, being present in 49% of medical students (n = 1428) according to a survey from several medical schools [2]. Urology residents (n = 211) identified dissatisfaction with their work-life balance as associated with increased burnout, an association with an odds ratio [OR] of 4.5, and a $p < 0.001$) [3]. The countries that participated were Portugal with a response rate of 30.5%, Italy with a response rate of 45.2%, USA with a response rate of 20.9%, Belgium with a response rate of 9.4%, and France with a response rate of 12.5%. Specifically, the respondents noted 'difficulty maintaining a relationship' and 'difficulty seeing friends and family'. These findings indicate poor time availability and inadequate relationship skills.

Individual Resilience

Programs to strengthen individual resilience have been in place for some time. The best of these programs focus on strengthening individual resilience through the use of peer support groups, time for reflection on patient care, mindfulness-based stress reduction, meditation promoting relaxation, and cognitive behavioral stress prevention exercises. Other training programs provide social support through interventions that bring trainees and their families together in informal gatherings.

The theoretical construct of resilience can be tied to specific educational approaches. For example, the development of self-efficacy requires less didactic and more self-directed learning. Coaching assumes that improvement is possible, and demonstrates that successful progression is based on persistence and commitment, as much as on innate ability and competitiveness. A synthesis of the nursing education literature on resilience summarizes the ideal education environment for developing professional resilience as one that establishes effective 'social connection with peers and other adults, positive role-modeling by winners or achievers, unobtrusive monitoring of well-being, and coaching to help in goal setting and elevating expectations' [4]. Many programs include the 'seeking of social support in an effective way'. Again, the process of seeking social support is not defined or described.

Individual resilience is also enhanced through formal changes to curricula and there is strong support for this endeavor, despite significant variation in studies such as when they are given, sample size, and outcome measures [5]. A systematic review of 21 studies of resilience curricula noted that the earliest study on resilience curricula in medical education was published in 1982, and that 90% have been published in the last decade. Interestingly, the comments of many study participants include comments about their families: "I just have the most supportive home environment imaginable and it's probably the major thing in my life that allows me to get through the weeks, so marry well."/"Just having someone not related to medicine that I can talk to … can be a big help." These comments point to the need to define and focus on relational resilience.

Further proof of the need for teaching and training in relational resilience is found in the interviews of 200 German physicians of different ages, disciplines, and hierarchical status. The study identified three dimensions of resilience strategies; (1) job-related gratifications derived from treatment interactions, (2) practices, such as leisure-time activities, self-demarcation, limitation of working hours, and continuous professional development, and (3) attitudes, such as acceptance of professional and personal boundaries, and a focus on positive aspects of work, and personal reflexivity [6]. Interviewees commented: 'Reliable family relations and friendships represented an oasis of stability and understanding. They provided relaxation through a change of focus and were beneficial for putting things in perspective. When my children say, "Mummy, you're hardly ever home these days," I know things are not as they should be. When I really am home and we do something together, I know that I can only communicate properly if I have reserves of strength. Whenever I'm on my last legs, I lose my bearings-at work as well.'

Physicians also reported that they found it helpful to have relationships with people who are prepared to bring them 'down to earth' when necessary. One commented 'It's important to find the right balance between self-overestimation and a lack of self-confidence. You need an environment of family and friends who will tell you when you start behaving badly. My wife is my severest critic.'

The cultivation of these relations normally took place in the framework of ritualized contexts e.g., going shopping together, sporting activities, lunch with the family, weekly meetings with friends in the local pub and via conscious presence e.g., 'When I'm home, I'm not anywhere else".

Relational Resilience

We are relational beings but there is sparse literature on how to understand and evaluate the relationships of healthcare trainees and professionals. The development of hope has been positively associated with physician wellbeing, and teaching modules developed for psychiatry trainees can be adapted for trainees [7, 8]. These modules improve trainees understanding of attachment, confiding, and embracing relationships. Trainees are encouraged to look for confiding or reconnecting relationships that provide intimate, "heart to heart" communion, attachment relationships that imbue confidence or a sense of security, adopting a good mentoring relationship, embracing or clarifying your role in a family, team, or work group, adding new members to your social networks that provide neighborly relationships characterized by reciprocal support, and the development of altruistic relationships that are generative in giving to others, perhaps helping someone who is facing similar difficulties. It is worth considering adding these modules to trainee curricula.

Digging deeper into the relationships of healthcare professionals, two prominent psychiatrists, Gabbard and Menninger held a retreat of 134 physicians and their spouses. They identified the role of the physician's compulsivity in their lives and their relationships [9]. They noted that these physicians had a marked discomfort with closeness, and a reluctance to acknowledge or address this. They also noted other aspects of compulsivity such as difficulty setting limits, chronic feelings that they are not doing enough, reluctance to take time away from work such as vacations, exaggerated sense of responsibility, self-doubt, guilt. These traits were displayed in a typical pattern with six features: erosion of marital intimacy, reduction of emotional expressiveness, absence of consistent and meaningful communication, and an avoidance of touchy subjects, limited sex, diversion of interests, mutual withdrawal ending in estrangement [9]. Again, it is worth considering exposing trainees to the idea that overcommitment to a professional identity might be at the expense of family relationships.

The emotional difficulties of coping with death and dying must also be considered for their impact on family relationships. These feelings of loss and grief may resonate with a trainee's own experiences of loss, and it is very helpful if this can be acknowledged. A lack of capacity to cope with loss can show up as detachment from others, and as emotional withdrawal from patients, colleagues, friends and family.

Framework for Understanding and Assessing the Health of Relationships

In this section I respond to the frequently noted comments that good social support and family support are key to trainee well-being and reduced burnout. I introduce several concepts from the family therapy literature to widen the scope of understanding and intervention. After introducing these concepts, I provide three case examples that show their application.

Understanding Family and Individual Life Cycles

The trainee is positioned in both the individual and family life cycle and discussion of this placement is a good entry into a discussion of relationships. Most trainees are in the early adulthood stage of the individual life cycle and in the early stages of the family life cycle. Chronic illnesses, second marriages, single parenthood are examples of deviations that impact the time line of the family stages. Extended time in training such as training in many of the healthcare disciplines, lengthens both the individual and family cycle stages, culminating in trainees trying to both train in their medical specialty and to establish a family, during the same critical time period. Many trainees, women especially, feel the pressure to have children before they are too old, and are usually faced with a training environment that is not that supportive. If the onus is placed on trainees to attend to their own health and relationships, the trainee may have to resist many of the structures of training, such as schedules, and the school time lines that are 'strongly encouraged'. The trainee may have to exert their desire to shape their career as they wish, over the needs of a supervisor who wants all trainees to move through the school's timeline efficiently.

The Individual Life Cycle

- Prebirth: Potential – The child who has not yet been born has unlimited potential
- Birth: Hope
- Infancy (Ages 0–3): Vitality
- Early Childhood (Ages 3–6): Playfulness
- Middle Childhood (Ages 6–8): Imagination
- Late Childhood (Ages 9–11): Ingenuity
- Adolescence (Ages 12–20): Passion
- Early Adulthood (Ages 20–35): Enterprise
- Midlife (Ages 35–50): Contemplation
- Mature Adulthood (Ages 50–80): Benevolence
- Late Adulthood (Age 80+): Wisdom
- Death & Dying: Life

The Family Life Cycle

- A committed couple
- Birth of a child
- Family with preschool kids
- Family with school-going kids
- Family with youngsters
- Family as launching centers
- Family in the middle years
- Aging family

Systems Thinking

Systems thinking is the core concept at the basis of all relational/family theory and intervention. Everyone exists in relationship and in a family system. When one person in the family has stress, this stress affects the rest of the family. Likewise, stress in the family affects each individual person. When discussing relationships, rather than thinking of social support, think about the family system and the impact of stress that reverberates through all the family members. It is a circular process that can feed on itself unless corrected. The stress of medical school affects everyone in the family and the stress needs to be addressed and managed by each family member. How well this stress is managed is reflected in the resilience inherent in the relationship/family.

Relational Resilience

Relational/family resilience has three overarching processes: communication, organization and a shared belief system [10]. Good communication means clear communication and the ability to communicate emotions with your partner/members of your family. Good organization means the ability to engage in collaborative adaptable problem-solving with your partner/family. Lastly a resilient family/relationship has a shared belief system, with shared ideas about meaning-making in the family, hope, and a shared spirituality. A shared spirituality means a shared set of beliefs that can be based on religion, or can be beliefs about the natural world, philantropy, teaching the next generation etc. This shared vision is a fundamental component of a successful relationship/family.

Dyadic Coping

Dyadic coping means that a couple copes as a unit. Any stress is viewed as 'our problem' and the couple work collaboratively on solving problems. Dyadic coping includes shared decision making about meals, exercise and schedules. Dyadic coping is reflected in the amount of 'we talk' the couple engages in. Questions such as 'How much do you want this to change?', can help clarify a couple's motivation to work together.

Self-Report Questionnaire

The Family Assessment Device (FAD) [11] is a commonly used self-report measure of family satisfaction or distress and is available in 27 languages (Table 7.1). The FAD is a 60-item tool that assesses family functioning across six dimensions; Roles, Communication, Problem solving, Emotional Involvement, Emotional Responsiveness, Behavior Control. It also contains a 12-item General Functioning Scale, the GF-FAD which is available on its own, and an ultra-brief version has been developed with three items (BAFFS), see Table 7.1 [12]. This tool can be used to identify strengths and weaknesses in relationships. The strengths in a relationship can be used to help the couple/family tackle their weaknesses. For example, if a couple is already good communicators about practical things, they can learn to communicate about their difficult emotions, using the same process of communication. If a couple are good individual problem solvers, they can learn to be good family problem solvers.

Table 7.1 Family Assessment Device

General Functioning Scale				
1. Planning family activities is difficult because we misunderstand each other.				
_______SA	_______A	_______D	_______SD	_________
2. In times of crisis we can turn to each other for support.				
_______SA	_______A	_______D	_______SD	_________
3. We cannot talk to each other about the sadness we feel.				
_______SA	_______A	_______D	_______SD	_________
4. Individuals are accepted for what they are.				
_______SA	_______A	_______D	_______SD	_________
5. We avoid discussing our fears and concerns.				
_______SA	_______A	_______D	_______SD	_________
6. We can express feelings to each other.				
_______SA	_______A	_______D	_______SD	_________
7. There are lots of bad feelings in the family.				
_______SA	_______A	_______D	_______SD	_________
8. We feel accepted for what we are.				
_______SA	_______A	_______D	_______SD	_________
9. Making decisions is a problem for our family.				
_______SA	_______A	_______D	_______SD	_________
10. We are able to make decisions about how to solve problems.				
_______SA	_______A	_______D	_______SD	_________
11. We don't get along well together.				
_______SA	_______A	_______D	_______SD	_________
We confide in each other.				
_______SA	_______A	_______D	_______SD	_________

SA strongly agree, *A* agree, *D* disagree, *SD* strongly disagree
Scoring for even numbered questions: SA = 1, A = 2, D = 3, SD = 4
Scoring for odd numbered questions is reverse scored. For each score as above, subtract from 5 to get the score. For example: 5–1 = 4
A resulting total of 2.00 or above, indicates problematic family functioning. The higher the score, the more problematic the person perceives their general family functioning
Epstein et al. [11]

Case Examples

Negotiating Clinical Rotations and Residency Placements

Krystal and Joe are in their early twenties and have been dating for 14 months. They have discussed marriage as a possible future option. Krystal is offered a prestigious training position on the West coast, which would involve 6 months apart. Joe is initially excited for her, but as the months go by, he sees her commitment to her career as off-putting and feels that he would always be in second place, behind her career. As their connection dwindles, Krystal begins to consider her options. She decides to quit her training and return home to marry Joe, feeling that she does not have 'the time or energy' to look for a new partner. Joe, on reflection of her sacrifice, decides that they need to be more thoughtful about their life together, otherwise resentments will drive them apart. Once married, they will seek opportunities that will only benefit them together, as a couple.

This means that both of them will sacrifice for the sake of the marriage, but neither will be the only person to sacrifice for the sake of the other. This means that both Krystal and Joe have to take into consideration if there are extended family members who might be able to help with childcare, or that they find childcare options in the community. They work hard at thinking through their difficulties and in the process, they develop relational resilience. They learn to communicate clearly and honestly, to organize their lives together and develop shared goals and a belief system about what is important to them.

Premarital Assessment

Josh and Sandra seek a couples assessment as part of their desire to make sure they understand their relationship prior to marriage. Josh is an emergency medicine resident. Sandra is a high school math teacher. At the assessment, Sandra's main complaint is that Josh is dismissive of her. She gives the example of being upset about something that happened in her classroom with two students. She wants to discuss it with Josh but he dismisses her.

Josh states "Her complaints are so trivial. I am dealing with life and death situations in the emergency room. Do you think I want to come home and listen to the squabbles between two teenagers that happened in her classroom?"

Sandra responds "These issues at school are important to me. If you dismiss them then you are dismissing me."

Josh retorts: "Well can you at least see my point of view?"

Sandra nods "Yes, but I feel that you dismiss me."

Josh retorts angrily "That is not my intention but do you have ANY IDEA what stress I am under at work?"

Sandra drops her head down and responds with a note of sadness, "Actually you don't talk about it, so I don't know."

The therapist asks how they would like to interact around their respective work stresses. The therapist models good listening behavior, giving each person an extended time to express their feelings without interruption. The therapist then gently asks the couple, "Do you want to listen to each other better? What is the point of sharing?"

Josh becomes reflective for the first time; "I am afraid of getting callous and losing my empathy. I see it in my colleagues, they say terrible things about patients sometimes. I don't want to be like that. I don't want to get burned out. I need Sandra. She helps bring balance into my life.".

Sandra responds quickly, "I am willing to help you but you must respect me. I know that I am not dealing with what you deal with, but my life is important to me, just as your life is important to you. You must accept that if we are to marry.'

Josh nods in agreement. After a short pause, the therapist follows up with "These are fine words and great sentiments, but what are you actually going to do that is different?"

The couple discusses this for a while and, with the therapists encouragement and coaching, they decide on several options to put into practice. They decided on the following:

1. When we come together at the end of the day, we will utilize relationship maintenance skills such as hugging, kissing, and touching each other. This can be as short as 5 min.
2. We will designate a time for each of us to discuss work issues. We agree on spending 10 min for each person, each night if needed, but at least once a week. We will check in each day to see if this time is needed.
3. We want our downtime together to be free of discussion of work difficulties.
4. Sandra will help Josh maintain his empathy for his patients and Josh will help Sandra with problem solving her issues at her job.

This couple came for two sessions. The first session consisted of an assessment which clarified their strengths and weaknesses. The second session consisted of the therapist coaching them in the relationship skills needed to pay attention to their goals and helped them find ways to resolve the issues that concerned them. The therapist did not suggest solutions but encouraged them to talk through options until they found solutions that they mutually agreed upon. A third session was scheduled for several months out to check on their progress. In summary, in two sessions, they learned to improve the resilience of their relationship by emotional sharing and collaborative problem solving. This case example shows how systems thinking is useful in clarifying the conflict: Josh and Sandra were initially unable to understand the role of their own stress on the other person.

When Different Values Collide and Break a Marriage

Priya got into medical school and got pregnant at the same time. It was not planned that way. Her spouse said Priya should stay home and take care of the baby. Priya felt conflicted but eventually asked the medical school if she could start a year later. This was granted. In the ensuing year, Priya looked after the baby and planned to start medical school when the baby was 1 year old. Her spouse and the spouse's family were outspoken in their opinion that she should not go to medical school, saying that she should stay home and care for the baby. They subtly equated going to medical school as being a neglectful mother. Priya was in a bind. It seemed to her that she would have to choose between her life dream of going to medical school or choose her marriage and the support of her in-laws. She chose medical school. Her spouse initiated divorce proceedings, angry and resentful that their opinion 'didn't seem to matter'. Priya's spouse stated that she never thought Priya would actually go to medical school, that it was just a pipe dream. Whatever the prior unspoken beliefs were, the couple divorced, leaving Priya as a part time single parent navigating medical school and tied to one town to avoid potential child custody issues. This marriage might have done well, if the individual and family life cycle stages had not clashed and their child had been born after training was completed.

Conclusion

Training as a healthcare professional occurs during the formative years of early adulthood. Healthcare trainees, especially physicians, have extraordinarily high self-expectations which make limitations in knowledge seem like a personal failing. Physicians act as though instant recall of facts is of particular importance. Medical training still emphasizes knowledge over the process of learning, and medical residents frequently express the belief that they don't read or know enough. Most find themselves disheartened when others quote articles they do not know on rounds or at morning report. They have not yet realized that learning is lifelong, facts change, and the ability to solve problems or find needed information is what matters. Physicians frequently have obsessive compulsive traits, which makes them good doctors, but can lead to a preference for work over family life. Medical marriages are often lived for the future, because the current perils of medicine take up the now.

Neglect of one's own self-care, one's health and one's relationships have, for too long, been the norm in healthcare. Steps are underway to change this, at an institutional level and at a personal level. Good social support is emphasized in studies of burnout and stress management but the concept of social support is without clear definition, and there is no clear understanding of how social support exists in relationships. The implication is that healthcare professionals should find an empathic partner, with little understanding of what the healthcare trainee brings to the relationship, both strengths and weaknesses.

An understanding of how to create resilient family relationships are vital for all families effective management of current and future stressors and major life events. Families with preexisting strengths in relationships can maintain closeness despite heightened family stress, and those who build resilience through good communication, organization and sharing of values and beliefs, will do better during the stressful experience of training. Preserving and/or building healthy family relationships will give family members, including children, the opportunity to thrive. We are relational beings and our interdependence is vital for our well-being and resilience.

Key Points

1. Be aware of signs and symptoms of burnout
2. Understand the role of the individual and family life cycles
3. Evaluate your relationship strengths and weaknesses with your partner/family so that you can develop preventative measures in your relationships.
4. Be proactive, using problem solving techniques, if problems arise.

Action Items

1. On acceptance into medical training, discuss in detail what the implications of the upcoming stressors will be with your spouse/partner/family.
2. If there are long standing relational difficulties such as communication difficulties or differences of opinion, for example when to start having children, address them fully. The goal is to tackle long standing difficulties before adding the stress of extended training at a critical individual and family life stage.
3. Work with your spouse/partner/family to be vigilant for signs of burnout and have a plan to address these signs. Make sure the plan includes the whole family.
4. Remember you are not alone. There are many of us who have trod this path before you. Reach out and ask for help. We have all received help and want to pass it on. Our interdependence is part of our well-being and resilience.

Thank you to Bella Curry, third year medical student at University of New England College of Osteopathic Medicine for providing suggestions and comments on this chapter.

References

1. Martin AR. Stress in residency. J Gen Intern Med. 1986;1:252–7.
2. Dyrbye LN, Moutier C, Durning SJ, et al. The problems program directors inherit: medical student distress at the time of graduation. Med Teach. 2011;33:756–8.
3. Marchali D, Goldman CC, Carvalho FFL, Talso M, Lynch JH, Esperto F, et al. Resident burnout in USA and European urology residents: an international concern. BJU Int. 2019;124(2):349–56.
4. Howe A, Smajdor A, Stockl A. Towards an understanding of resilience and its relevance to medical training. Med Educ. 2012;46(4):349–56.
5. Seo C, Corrado M, Fournier K, Bailey T, Haykal KA. Addressing the physician burnout epidemic with resilience curricula in medical education: a systematic review. BMC Med Educ. 2021;21(1):80.
6. Zwack J, Schweitzer J. If every fifth physician is affected by burnout, what about the other four? Resilience strategies of experienced physicians. Acad Med. 2013;88(3):382–9.
7. Huber A, Strecker C, Kachel T, Höge T, Höfer S. Character strengths profiles in medical professionals and their impact on well-being. Front Psychol. 2020;11:566728.
8. Griffith JL. Hope modules: brief psychotherapeutic interventions to counter demoralization from daily stressors of chronic illness. Acad Psychiatry. 2018;42:135–45.
9. Gabbard GO, Menninger RW. The psychology of postponement in the medical marriage. JAMA. 1989;261:2378–81.
10. Walsh F. Strengthening family resilience. New York, NY: Guilford Press; 2015.
11. Epstein NB, Baldwin LM, Bishop DS. The McMaster family assessment device. J Marital Fam Ther. 1983;9(2):171–80.
12. Mansfield AK, Keitner GI, Sheeran T. The brief assessment of family functioning scale (BAFFS): a three-item version of the general functioning scale of the family assessment device. Psychother Res. 2019;29(6):824–31.

Strategies & Tactics to Support a High Performing Healthcare Workforce

8

Elizabeth Harry and Richard Joseph

Provider Burnout

The epidemic of burnout among physicians has come into national spotlight in recent years and has been further magnified by the COVID-19 pandemic. Burnout is a long-term stress reaction defined by a clinical syndrome of emotional exhaustion, depersonalization, and a lack of sense of personal accomplishment.[1]

The prevalence of burnout amongst physicians and health care providers is alarmingly high. At any given time in any given medical and surgical specialty, one in three physicians is experiencing burnout. An online survey of 15,000 doctors finds an overall physician burnout rate of 42%.[2] The study found that 43.9% of U.S. physicians exhibited at least one symptom of burnout in 2017.[3] Notably, women have consistently reported higher percentages of burnout then men. And several studies have also found a high prevalence of burnout and depression among trainees—medical students and residents [1, 2].

The burnout symptoms experienced by individual clinicians are the result of a systemic disease. Being a physician is an inherently stressful job. Dealing with sick, hurt, and dying patients is an emotionally intense and exacting responsibility. Throughout the course of our professional development, most physicians develop the strategies to cope with this stress. But given the baseline nature of the job,

[1] https://www.who.int/news/item/28-05-2019-burn-out-an-occupational-phenomenon-international-classification-of-diseases

[2] https://www.medscape.com/slideshow/2020-lifestyle-burnout-6012460?faf=1

[3] https://www.mayoclinicproceedings.org/article/S0025-6196(18)30938-8/fulltext

E. Harry (✉)
University of Colorado School of Medicine, UCHealth, Aurora, CO, USA
e-mail: ELIZABETH.HARRY@CUANSCHUTZ.EDU

R. Joseph
Harvard Medical School, Brigham and Women's Hospital, Boston, MA, USA

© The Author(s), under exclusive license to Springer Nature Switzerland AG 2022

P. K. Louie et al. (eds.), *The Successful Health Care Professional's Guide*,
https://doi.org/10.1007/978-3-030-95950-0_8

physicians are naturally more susceptible to excess stress, which, if unremitting, can cause burnout. And in the modern health care delivery environment, sources of excess stress are ubiquitous.

Drivers of Burnout

The current drivers of burnout can be understood on the continuum from the macro the personal level.

Organizational Factors

At the level of the health care system, physicians are increasingly inundated with administrative tasks and bureaucratic hoops, which are epitomized by the labyrinthine and duplicative data entry in electronic health records. The complexity of care itself is also increasing exponentially as medical knowledge advances. The clerical burden and complexity of care contribute to an excessive workload with long hours, time pressure, and a lack of control.

At the organizational level, many physicians feel affronted by an unfavorable and even noxious work culture. In business and management, it is widely known that one's work satisfaction and stress levels are directly impacted by the leadership skills of the immediate supervisor. Unsurprisingly, the same is true for physician job satisfaction [3]. And yet leadership and management training is not typically included as a core competency in our professional development. This psychic toll of poor leadership can compound other job-related stresses including call schedules, compensation formulas, organizational politics, personality clashes, etc.

Personal and Societal Factors

Despite popular cultural portrayals which convey the opposite, physicians are not impervious to stresses outside of the work environment. Cultural shifts have changed the nature and expectation of work in the modern era. And the demographics of the modern physician workforce have changed as well with women now representing over one third of the physician workforce.[4] Many physicians are saddled with debt from their years of education. And many physicians are juggling dual career households with children and seemingly endless responsibilities outside of work.

Impact of Training

And finally, let's not forget the training process itself. Our training teaches us the exact opposite of how to sustain ourselves and recharge. We learn (and are often encouraged) to ignore our own physical, emotional, and spiritual needs in service of patient care and in fear of appearing weak, unenthused, or even uncommitted. Traits like workaholism, perfectionism, self-denial, and independence help us get into medical school and stand out amongst our peers; naturally, they become hard wired.

[4] https://www.aamc.org/data-reports/workforce/interactive-data/active-physicians-sex-and-specialty-2019

However, these once adaptive behavior patterns soon become maladaptive and set us up for burnout. Additionally, the hierarchical nature of medical training instills a learned helplessness and conditions a lack of agency, which now underlies many practicing physicians' feelings of professional dissatisfaction and burnout.[5]

The combined impact of these and other factors causes what Christina Maslach, preeminent authority on occupational burnout and creator of the Maslach Burnout Inventory [4], describes as "an erosion of the soul caused by a deterioration of one's values, dignity, spirit, and will" [5].

The consequences, for both physicians and their patients, are dire. The health of burned-out physicians suffer [6] with higher rates of alcohol and drug misuse [7], depression [8], and suicidality [9, 10]. Burnout has a deleterious impact on the safety, access, and quality of health care [11]. Suffering physicians are more likely to leave clinical practice [12, 13] which reduces access to care. The quality of care suffers as depersonalization leads to poor interactions with patients [14]. Burned-out physicians experience impaired attention, memory, and executive function which threatens patient safety, increases medical errors [15], and heightens malpractice risk.

Physician burnout also has imperative financial implications for health care institutions—it is costly! Approximately $4.6 billion per year is lost in direct cost secondary to physician burnout, with the greatest proportion coming from physician turnover. For an organization, the cost of burnout is about $7600 per physician per year due to the resultant reduction in professional effort and loss of productivity [16]. The costs to replace one physician depends on specialty, location, and length of vacancy, with estimated costs ranging from hundreds of thousands to more than $1 million [17, 18]. Hence, there is not only a moral, but an economic imperative for leaders of health care provider systems to invest in the wellbeing and sustained performance of the physician workforce.

Strategies to Address Burnout

Recognizing and measuring physician burnout is a critical first step in the effort to manage an epidemic that has already spread. Thankfully, many large health care institutions have recognized the problem and have put resources towards assessing the workload and satisfaction levels of their physicians. In 2016, chief executives from 10 major health care organizations committed to 11 actions, including measuring physician well-being, supporting models of care that allow physicians to operate at the top of their license, and proactively monitoring and addressing the increasing regulatory burden imposed on physicians [19]. Current strategies to address burnout fall into two main categories: physician directed interventions focusing on individuals and organizational or structural directed interventions directed at the work environment.

[5] https://catalyst.nejm.org/doi/full/10.1056/CAT.18.0283

Individual Interventions

On the individual level, medical school and residency programs focus predominantly on providing the clinical knowledge and managing the clerical burden of providing medical care in the modern health care system. Despite the high level of burnout and depression amongst trainees, most programs do not provide the necessary learnings and practices for how to manage oneself and others in what has become a complex and stressful health care environment. Often, medical school and post-graduate programs sprinkle in some "wellness" offerings like yoga and ice cream socials into jam packed curricula and largely inflexible schedules. Some practicing physicians have access to mindfulness training, stress management, and cognitive behavioral techniques to enhance job competence and improve communication skills and personal coping strategies. Some of these programs have promising results and improve physician coping strategies [20–22]. Unsurprisingly, however, the organization-directed interventions are generally associated with a more meaningful reduction in burnout [23].

Many healthcare organizations preach the importance of boosting physician resiliency. Resilience describes "the ability of an individual to respond to stress in a healthy, adaptive way such that personal goals are achieved at minimal psychological and physical cost; resilient individuals not only 'bounce back' rapidly after challenges but also grow stronger in the process."[6] Although efforts to maintain or strengthen resilience are appropriate, increasing resilience amongst physicians is often and infuriating proposition as it falsely implies a baseline deficiency of it.[7] Selling resilience as a form of personal nourishment puts the responsibility for change firmly on the individual. Equal or greater emphasis must be placed on addressing characteristics of the practice and regulatory environments that contribute to burnout.[8] While resilience training may be helpful in addressing unavoidable suffering, it is the wrong treatment for the organizational pathologies that lead to avoidable suffering.

Organizational Interventions

Many institutions have developed wellbeing models to help define what factors must be attended to when developing strategic plans for attention to wellbeing [24]. The National Academy of Medicine recommends a focus on a combination of individually and institutionally owned domains, such as individual skills, personal factors, society and culture, rules and regulations, organizational factors, learning and practice environment, and health care responsibilities. Tait Shanafelt and colleagues describe 9 factors that, when optimized, lead to engagement and when not optimized, can lead to burnout [25]. These domains are workload and job demands, control and flexibility, work-life integration, social and community support at work, organizational culture and values, and efficiency and resources. Notably, in each

[6] https://journals.lww.com/academicmedicine/fulltext/2013/03000/Physician_Resilience___What_It_Means,_Why_It.12.aspx

[7] https://jamanetwork.com/journals/jamanetworkopen/fullarticle/2767829

[8] https://jamanetwork.com/journals/jamanetworkopen/fullarticle/2767829

domain, there are ways individuals, teams, work units, institutions, and regulatory bodies can have impact. Each educational and health care organization needs to decide for itself which domains are most important and complete and needs assessment and gap analysis to identify which next steps to take in order to most optimize the system with which they work. Key to each of these domains, however, is the need to focus on the way we complete work and the health and efficiency of our teams as we do so. Each moment we spend on unnecessary tasks is a moment wasting our most valuable resource: time.

The Current State

Current approaches to burnout focus on management rather than prevention. Much like the health care systems approach to intervening only when patients are sick, we currently approach physician burnout reactively and treat the symptoms of burnout with bandages and anesthetics. In order to determine a more proactive and preventive approach that empowers physician to thrive, it is useful to dig a layer deeper into the current experience of most physicians in the modern health care delivery environment.

What Providers Experience

As self-determination theory suggests, individuals are motivated to grow and change when their needs for competence, connection, and autonomy are fulfilled.[9] Physicians are an especially intrinsically motivated group who spend years of dedicated training in order to develop the skillset and authority to provide excellent patient care. It comes as no surprise, then, that physicians find meaning in their work when they are able to practice and deliver this skillset to with a sense of sense of autonomy, flexibility, and control.[10] The practice of medicine is predicated on having requisite time and focused attention to perform optimally—whether that be empathetically listening to a patient or performing a complex surgery. Continued learning and refinement of this skillset encourages mastery, which is intrinsically rewarding. The connection to patients who are benefiting from this practice, and colleagues who are sharing in this unique experience of caregiving fuels a sense of connection and reinforces a sense of professional purpose.

The values and motivators of many physicians are currently misaligned with those of the health care industry in which they work. Providing excellent patient care is often at odds with the incentives and imperatives of insurance companies, pharmacies, the hospital and clinic administrators. Financial imperatives for

[9] https://www.springer.com/gp/book/9780306420221

[10] https://www.ama-assn.org/practice-management/physician-health/magnificent-7-these-are-keys-boosting-physician-well-being

standardization, cost controls and productivity targets can all conflict with what is best for the patient and infringe on a physician's hard-earned expertise and judgement.

Time for meaningful work and collegiality is scarce in today's healthcare environment. Growing laws, regulations, and administrative requirements interfere with patient care and "drain time and morale" from physicians. Multiple sources of documentation requirements lead to duplicative and inconsistent requirements that are burdensome and time consuming for physicians. Many performance measures are not clinically relevant. Prior authorization rules for various medications and diagnostics vary by different payers, which require inconsistent workflow processes and submission of additional information through a manual process. Physicians must complete maintenance of certification (MOC) requirements because it is typically handled after work. And in our increasingly litigious environment, all physicians face the omnipresent threat of malpractice lawsuits. All of these external stresses strain a physician's ability to do meaningful work and impair connectedness amongst colleagues.

The Science Behind the Experience

Ultimately, we experience our lives based on where we focus our attention. Given the unyielding external stresses and distractions in today's health care environment, a deeper understanding of the mechanics of attention can inform our understanding of the current struggles and provide insights for potential solutions to enhance provider wellbeing and fulfillment.

Fundamentally, all that is learned or acted on from learning is processed through short term working memory, a finite resource [26]. Working memory has been described as "… a temporary storage system under attentional control that underpins our capacity for complex thought" [27]. Understanding this sentence is critical to understand the use of the limited resource we possess with which to do our complex work.

The finite working memory we all have can be depleted in a predictable way, and can be restored, when used properly. Cognitive Load Theory describes the way in which working memory is used or depleted [28]. This depletion depends on three factors: how complex the task at hand is (intrinsic load), how much working memory must be devoted to learning or creating mental models of the task at hand (germane load), and how much extraneous working memory must be used to collect the necessary data for and focus on the task at hand (extraneous load). The combination of these three factors depletes our working memory and, when overloaded, can lead to a process of load shedding, or data loss, that leads to lost information and risk of error [29]. Notably, working memory can recover with rest [30], meaning that taking a break between cognitively demanding tasks can allow recovery of this finite resource to begin a new cognitively demanding task at full capacity. Understanding these two fundamental points about how our brains process information is key when we attempt to educate learners in an ever more complex environment about ever more complex topics and when we try to complete our tasks in environments with increasing distraction (extraneous cognitive load) and harried pace (reducing the ability for restoration of cognitive resources).

Understanding the mechanics of attention is not only important to ensure proper attention is given to creating environments optimal for learning and patient care, but also to ensure the wellbeing of the entire healthcare team. Physicians reporting higher levels of task load also reported higher rates of burnout [31]. There are increasing calls to respond to the impact of divided attention in the healthcare space, defining team norms and expectations, workflows, and workspaces to optimize cognitive processing [32]. Specifically, the multitasking culture adopted throughout our society, including in the halls of our graduate schools and hospitals, leads to increasing mistakes and information overload [33]. Most critically, however, is the simple fact that where we place our attention, our energy and focus follow. Where we place our energy and focus is where, when compounded over years, we spend the energy of our lives. Often, with such a reactive culture surrounding attention placement, we give the guiding reigns of our focus away to whatever most urgently demands our attention, even if this is not what is most important to us in our lives, or where we would like to spend our time. Skills in defining one's values and priorities, while being able to place boundaries and restrictions around the ever-present siren call of distractors, will be even more critical as complexity increases. Coaching is one mechanism to help individuals gain these skills and keep them top of mind as they navigate their training.

Future State: Empowering Providers for High Performance

Tackling systemic reform to reduce regulatory requirements and reinstate a sense of autonomy among medical professionals is essential. At the same time, we must do more to help physicians manage themselves, lead teams, and shape organizational culture in an inherently stressful and increasingly complex health care environment. We should be engaging physicians in an ongoing professional (and personal) development curriculum that provides the training, tactics, and tools for high performance.

Consider how you would design healthcare education or delivery if you built it now, from the ground up, with the knowledge we have today. The science of performance psychology, cognitive load, and team dynamics and organizational culture arms us with all we need to build the health care education and delivery of the future. This future state would focus on 4 interrelated key principles (Fig. 8.1) and examples of each tactic at the individual and organizational level are described in Table 8.1.

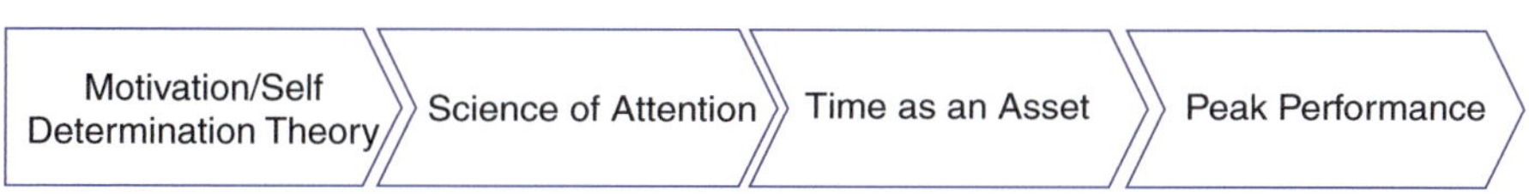

Fig. 8.1 4 Principles for high performing providers

Table 8.1 The 4 principles for high performing providers with representative examples and sub-components of each at individual team/org systems level

	Individual	Individual as organizational leader and change agent
Foster intrinsic motivation	Values assessment Personal coaching Gratitude practices Reflecting on individual mission, vision, and values	Salary based reimbursement. Avoid RVU or incentive based reimbursement. Diversify role types to meet many types of interests and allow individuals to craft jobs that fit their interests and skill sets Create time for the development of competence in a craft
Enhance attention & focus	Personal coaching Awareness training Time blocking, Pomodoro timing Discussions with teams regarding interruptions	Focus work spaces Agreements of what warrants interruptions on a care team
Honor time as a non-renewable asset	Personal coaching Time/value analysis Time blocking/ Pomodoro blocks Schedule high priority items into the week first Schedule personal priorities on your calendar	Evaluate team structure and delivery of care models Consider pyramid care delivery models that enhance the ability of each team member to deliver care. Examples were found during COVID of several physician assistants reporting to hospitalists who reported to an intensivist to spread the impact of the intensivist [34].
Train for peak performance	Personal ergonomic analysis	Offerings to support development of peak performance

Principle 1:
Foster Intrinsic Motivation: Engage in work primarily because it is personally rewarding as an opportunity to explore learn and actualize one's potential; not for an external reward.

Principle 2:
Enhance Attention & Focus: Use the science of cognitive processing, attention, and errors while multitasking to develop systems and workflows that optimize focused attention.

Principle 3:
Honor Time as a Non-renewable Asset: Time is our most valuable resource and we must practice treating it as such.

Principle 4:
Train for Peak Performance: Put your mind and body in a ready state to achieve optimal outcomes or performance of a given task in a consistent and sustainable manner

Discussion of the 4 Principles

Principle 1—Foster Intrinsic Motivation

Self Determination Theory has long told us that the internalization and integration of tasks depends on the degree to which the task is undertaken due to internal motivators such as relatedness, competence, and autonomy, or external factors such as demands, rewards and punishment. The more intrinsically motivated a task is, the more commitment there is from the participant in the completion of the task. Any system that focuses on extrinsic motivation is going against decades of research in the theories of motivation. Examples include grades, monetary incentives including RVU based incentives. In fact, RVU based incentives have been associated with higher rates of burnout.

It is due to the impact of this intrinsic motivation that it is key to know what one's values and purpose are. Values are at the core of our identity; we work to make sure our actions align with our values; when they do not, this causes internal tension and conflict. Our purpose is our why; how we hope to contribute to the world. This is the key for resiliency during challenging times.

Coaching is a key technique that can help individuals identify their values and their purpose as well as define and build skills in order to maintain intrinsic motivation. It is key to differentiate coaching from mentorship and sponsorship. Mentorship is the act of a senior member of the field teaching junior members how to complete a certain process or how to navigate a certain career. Sponsorship is the act of exchanging political capital for the advancement of a sponsee. This can come in the form of connecting, opportunity giving, or advocating. King on the other hand, believes that the answers to navigate one's careers are already within the individual. The coach helps the individual move from where they are to where they would like to be as defined by the individual. A coach, therefore, does not need to have training in the same field of study as the individual they are coaching. Mentorship has long been a tradition in healthcare education. Coaching and sponsorship are emerging as critical adjuncts to mentorship with coaching linked to significant decreases in burnout and sponsorship linked to significant improvement in professional advancement.

Key aspects of coaching include identifying limiting and strengthening thoughts, behaviors, and action patterns, aiding participants in moving from their current state to their desired state and advising regarding best practices. Increasingly, randomized studies are demonstrating that formal coaching programs decrease burnout not only in the recipient of the coaching, but also in those trained to deliver the coaching. In the upcoming section we will highlight three example case studies.

Case Study: Valor Performance

Since 2018, a leading academic medical center located in Boston has partnered with Valor Performance[11] to offer an innovative performance coaching program to support physician leadership development and improve well-being. The virtual program utilizes structured interactions with a professionally trained performance coach complemented by a digital curriculum focusing on emotional intelligence, communication, time and energy management, confidence, and aligning personal values with professional duties.

After the launch of the program, the medical center received 120 applications within one week and identified an initial cohort of 40 female physicians and faculty to pilot in their inaugural coaching program. The program was later expanded to an additional 115 male and female faculty within the first year, and an additional 160 physicians the following year. Each participant received ten 45-minute professional coaching sessions across a six-month period, weekly evidenced-based digital exercises, and unlimited access to a learning library of self-directed content.

The success of the initial program was assessed in pre- and post-surveys that employ validated instruments, as well as through qualitative measures such as engagement rates and net promoter score (See Exhibit). The data-driven results from Valor Performance include improvements across work engagement, optimism levels, and perceived stress levels, with perceived stress levels having the largest change from baseline with an average decrease of 29%. Lagging indicators also suggest a correlation between the coaching program and physician retention. Despite recent survey data indicating that 54% of U.S. physicians have changed their employment plans due to COVID-19 [35], the organization has retained 83% of the physicians in the initial cohort.

> *"I started this coaching program with no idea what to expect, and at a pretty low point in my career.* ***I was completely burnt out from my experience of the covid surge, I did not have a clear career path forward, and I was starting to look for other jobs.*** *[My Coach] helped me to re-define my values and career goals.* ***I received a new promotion and non-clinical time to support my roles. [My Coach] has helped me develop valuable leadership skills for my new role as fellowship program director."***

[11] Valor Performance was founded in 2017 by CEO Sarah Milby, and utilizes the latest research in performance and positive psychology, as well as the best practices of elite athletes to support high-performing professionals in optimizing their mental game and mindset for success. Valor coaches are experts in performance psychology, behavioral psychology, organizational development and related fields and 50% are world-class high performers themselves, including Olympians paralympians and former elite military leaders.

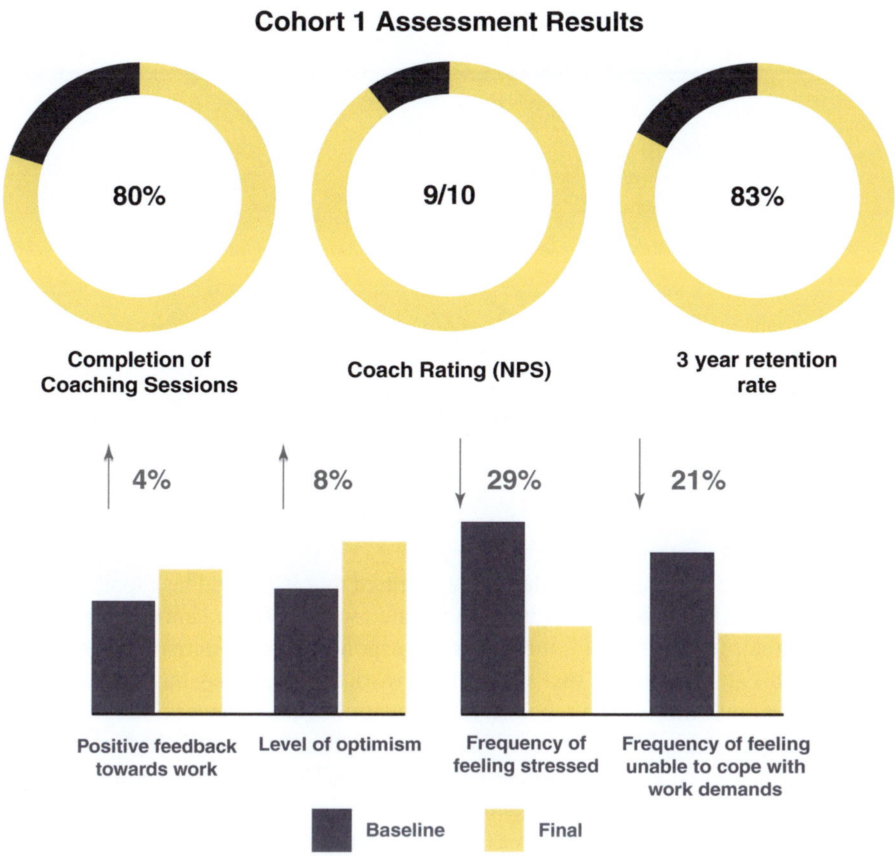

Principle 2–Science of Attention

Attention describes the sustained focus of cognitive resources on information while filtering or ignoring extraneous information. Focus, the ability to control and direct one's attention towards an important task, is foundational for job satisfaction.

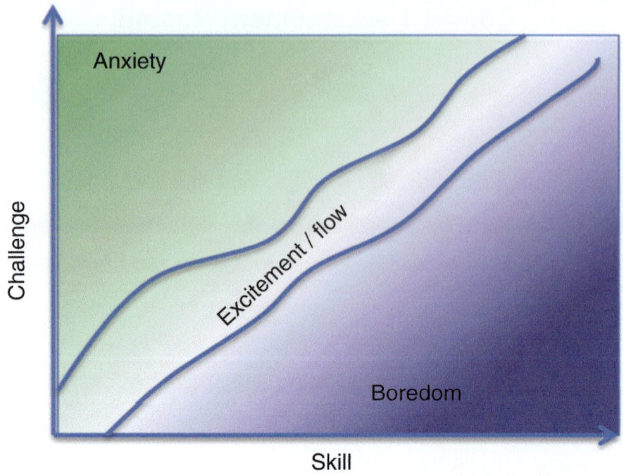

Ref: Mihaly Csikszentmihalyi

Human Factors Evaluations

Recently, a large national survey has demonstrated that increased task load, as measured by the NASA Task Load Index is associated with increased burnout. For every 10 point increase in task load, there is a corresponding 33% increase in reporting burnout. This study suggests that attending to work task load may have an impact in reducing burnout. Many high reliability organizations focus on workload reduction. This can be done through process improvement methods such as LEAN methodology or evaluation by experts such as Human Factor Engineers and Organizational Psychologists. Utilizing resources and expertise to redesign work environments for focused attention is critical to allow peak performance. When people are allowed to focus, they can enter a state of flow and create incredibly high quality work.

Flow

As originally described by psychologist Mihaly Csikszentmihalyi, "flow" is "a state in which people are so involved in an activity that nothing else seems to matter; the experience is so enjoyable that people will continue to do it even at great cost, for the sheer sake of doing it". Known colloquially as being "in the zone," flow is characterized by present moment concentration on a singular task, a clear objective with immediate feedback, a sense of effortlessness and control, and an absence of time and self-consciousness. In essence, flow is characterized by the complete absorption in what one does, and a resulting transformation in one's sense of time. Flow happens within that narrow window between boredom and anxiety where the perceived challenge matches one's current skill level.

We tend associate stress with distress—when you feel overwhelmed because your resources (physically, mentally, emotionally) are inadequate to meet the demands you're facing. However, there is also eustress. Eustress is usually a product of nerves, which can be brought on when faced with a fun challenge. Eustress helps us stay motivated, work toward goals, and feel good about life. Eustress is all about sufficiently challenging yourself without expending all your resources. Eustress focuses our attention and make us feel alive, excited, and engaged.

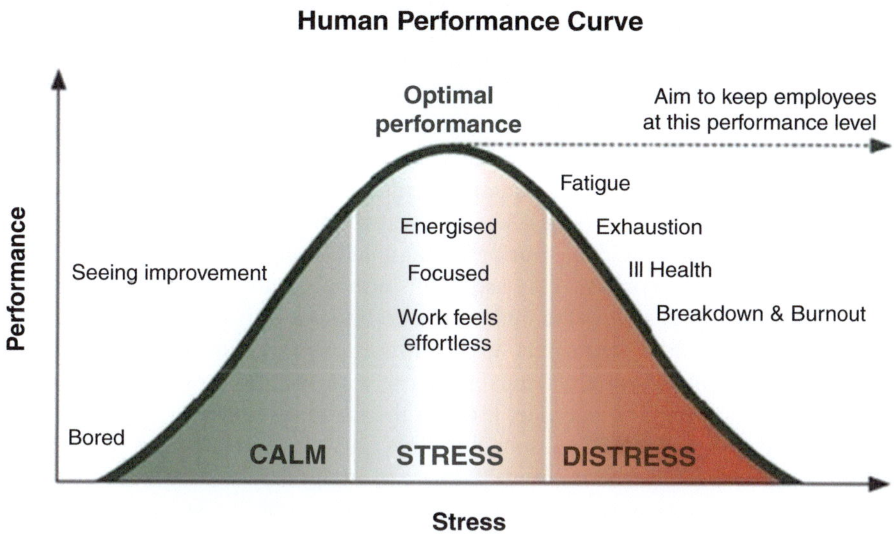

Although the specifics of the Yerkes-Dobson Law are under debate in more recent research,[12] the Human Performance and Stress Curve remains instructive. A certain level of stress is actually necessary to enhance our focus and attention. Performance is a function of the severity and duration of this stress. Too little arousal doesn't provide much in the way of motivation. Too much arousal causes a stronger stress reaction that can hamper performance. There is a zone where we feel motivated and energized with just enough discomfort and stimulation without tipping over to feeling overwhelmed and exhausted. That optimal level of arousal differs from person to person, according to factors like the specific task, degree of skill, and confidence level. Too much stress destroys our ability to focus and, if unremitting, can lead to fatigue, exhaustion, and burnout.

Ultimately, we need to find that healthy balance of eustress for optimal performance at work and in life. Eustress is a necessary trigger for personal development, which in intrinsically rewarding. But we must grow slowly, deliberately, and carefully. We are not designed to handle a stressful stimulus for too long. We can only grow if we pair a stressful stimulus with adequate rest and recovery. In their book "Peak Performance" Brad Stuhlberg and Steve Magness offer this simple, yet powerful equation: Stress + Rest = Growth.[13] This is why recovery is an essential component of a training program for peak performance (see section "Principle 4—Train for Peak Performance").

[12] https://ntrs.nasa.gov/citations/20060017835

[13] https://www.amazon.com/Peak-Performance-Elevate-Burnout-Science/dp/162336793X

Principle 3–Time as an Asset

In addition to attention being an unrenewable asset, time is an often-unrecognized non-renewable asset. Most of our assets can be renewed. If we lose money this can be regenerated. If we lose material goods, these can be replaced. The draw on our attention, however, cannot be replaced in as much as it takes our time away from other potentially more valuable areas where we may be able to focus our attention. While we can restore our working memory through breaks, we can never recuperate the lost time spent focusing on distracting items.

Recognizing we are building a knowledge economy where we depend on the knowledge individuals cultivate during training and healthcare education, we must value the asset of their time and the use of this non-renewable source of knowledge above all other assets as it is the most resource limited. This is not how we inherently think about valuing our assets. In fact, monetary asset acquisition often drives attention away from tasks most critical for those with specific skill sets to be spending their attention on. For example, often in the name of efficiency, highly skilled physicians may find themselves spending time on tasks that could be easily completed by someone with less training. To move to an optimal training and care delivery environment, we must honor time as an unrenewable resource and be very careful with how we use the asset of those who have built the ability to contribute to a knowledge economy.

During Covid, many novel systems were built that allowed one physician to extend to see many more patients, using their time more effectively through pyramid structures of evaluation and reporting [36]. There are infinite possibilities of how care delivery can be structured to maximize the things we value most, from patient safety and patient experience to ability for care providers to have focused attention and time to think critically about the care they are providing. Taking our attention and time into account allows us to set up the environment for peak performance.

Principle 4—Train for Peak Performance

Meeting our high professional standards day in and day out requires systematic and intentional training. Whereas stress management is defensive and reactive, performance is offensive and preemptive. Depression screenings and mental health resources help with coping, whereas performance training optimizes for thriving. A campaign against burnout combats dis-ease, whereas a curriculum for performance promotes vitality. Performance is immediate and tangible, whereas wellness is delayed gratification — a notoriously hard sell. Building a new skill set in personal performance to enhance both self- and patient care generates an internal locus of control, which drives motivation and action.

We must provide health care professionals with the principles and opportunities to practice behaviors that maintain our energy, manage ourselves, and continually grow in an inherently stressful work environment. Resilience demands a dedicated curriculum and supported practice engaging with a sometimes harsh reality. Consider training in the military, which is a comparable hierarchical system with a rigorous and top-down training process U.S. soldiers now participate in a formal Comprehensive Soldier Fitness program,[14] a key component of which features Master Resilience Training.[15] A proactive strategy to prevent post-traumatic stress disorder, this curriculum has been called the "backbone of a cultural transformation of the U.S. Army in which a psychologically fit army will have equal standing with a physically fit army" [37]. More than 95% of participants attest to using these skills both on the job and in their personal lives [38].

Physicians, like the armed forces, business executives, and Olympic athletes, need coaches, drills, and routines to develop heightened self-awareness, better emotional regulation, healthier routines, and restorative practices—the skillset to stay on top of their game. Key principles, which are discussed in depth below or in other chapters throughout this text, include:

- physiology optimization
- self-awareness & mindset
- goal setting (See Chap. 4)
- habit formation
- deliberate practice for technical skill development (see Chap. 3)
- perseverance and grit (see Chap. 2)
- Self-compassion & spirituality

Physiology Optimization

Health care provider groups and delivery systems must think critically about having an ongoing curriculum to teach and support the behaviors that optimize physiology and help providers sustain focus, energy, and attention. This includes proper sleep, sustenance, movement, and recovery. Underinvesting in these foundational factors in human performance is underinvesting in the human capital that drives results for healthcare delivery systems. See Table 8.2 for sample solutions that might be part of a comprehensive physiology optimization plan for a group of high performing physicians.

Self-Awareness & Mindset

It was Aristotle who said "Knowing yourself is the beginning of all wisdom." Many spiritual teachers would argue that this is the essence of consciousness—what makes us unique as human beings. Our thought patterns—many of which become habitual over time—fuel emotions which can cause immense suffering. As human beings, we have the power to step away from our thoughts and observe them as they are generated in real time. We can choose not to identify with our thoughts and look at them without bias or judgement. And if we learn how to do this and practice it, we become more aware of ourselves, our tendencies, our habits, and why we do

[14] https://www.usar.army.mil/CSF/

[15] https://www.usar.army.mil/MRT/

Table 8.2 Sample curriculum for physiology optimization

Domain	Tests/trackers	Techniques	Tools	Team
Sleep	Polysomnogram; wearable sleep devices	Sleep efficiency	Access to call rooms, nap pods; blackout curtains and white noise machines	Sleep therapists
Sustenance	Food logs; continuous glucose monitors	How to strategically use food as fuel	Access to high energy snacks; recipes for quick and healthy meals; local meal delivery services	Nutritionists
Movement	CV capacity and stamina; pedometers	Workout plans and scheduling	Standing desks, access to on site fitness facilities; discounted gym memberships and virtual fitness offerings	Personal trainers; physical therapists; postural specialists
Recovery	Heart rate variability monitors; subjective assessments	Meditation, breath work	Work rooms with sunlight exposure and plants & biophilic design, quiet rooms	Psychologists

what we do. And if we can understand why we do what we do, we can challenge self-defeating beliefs that are not aligned with our desired values and self.

Awareness is the first step. Self-awareness is the ability to consciously monitor our thoughts, emotions, and beliefs in real time. Certain tools can help surface and magnify the thoughts and beliefs that may be holding us back in our life and causing suffering. They include:

1. Mindful meditation: Mindful meditation is all about cultivating this "awakening" or "awareness" in the present moment so that we can observe our thoughts non-judgmentally and learn about the inner workings of our mind. In the practice, the breath generally serves as an anchor point for our attention. During the practice, it is normal for our brain to do what it does best—to create thoughts that pop into our head that then create emotions that hook our attention. Or we may become distracted by body sensations, sounds around us, etc. The practice is learning how to recognize when we become distracted, when our mind wanders, and gently bring it back to the breath. With practice you become more aware of your thoughts as they arise, you learn to dissociate your "self" from your thoughts, your focus and attention improve, and you get better at self-regulation.
2. Journaling: a blank page provides a mechanism for us to get thoughts out of our minds. When the thoughts are out of our mind, they tend to have less influence on our emotions and we can look at them more objectively.
3. Reading: Reading books, particularly philosophical texts or fictional works that portray the shared human experience, can teach us more about ourselves and our own journey.

4. Therapy: having a trained professional listen to us and reflect our thoughts back to us is another way for us to get a distanced, objective view on our own thoughts. Unfortunately, therapy still carries a stigma, but it can be a powerful tool for us to view, organize, and challenge our thoughts with the help of an unbiased secondary party.

William James, known as the father of modern psychology, once said that "Human beings can alter their lives by altering their attitudes of mind." Cognitive behavioral therapy (CBT) is predicated on this awareness of mind. It focuses on challenging and changing unhelpful cognitive distortions (e.g. thoughts, beliefs, and attitudes) and behaviors, improving emotional regulation, and the development of personal coping strategies that target solving current problems. Traditionally, CBT is applied to specific conditions like depression, anxiety, substance use disorders, etc. But the principles of CBT can be applied and are helpful for helping with behavior change in any realm of life and how to better manage stressful life situations.

First you identify some challenging situation, difficulty, or condition that you are facing in your life. Once you have done this, the key first step is to identify your thought patterns. The second step is to examine your thoughts. Ask yourself whether your view of a situation is based on fact or on an inaccurate perception of what's going on. And finally, CBT usually involves efforts to change behavioral patterns such as using positive affirmations or using role playing to prepare for potentially problematic interactions with others. In essence, CBT helps you become aware of inaccurate or negative thinking so you can view challenging situations more clearly and respond to them in a more effective way.

Our mindset, the frame of mind through which we perceive, interpret, and organize an inherently complex world, has a direct and measurable effect on our health and wellbeing. Our mindset shapes our reality by influencing attention, affect, motivation, and physiology. In her groundbreaking book "Mindset," Carol Dweck reveals that the way we view our own intelligence has a strong influence on our success.[16] A fixed mindset is a belief that talents and abilities are set-in-stone. If you have this mindset, you may feel that you hold a certain amount of intelligence, perhaps offered by genetics or circumstances, and nothing can be done to alter it. You may find yourself becoming preoccupied with proving your talents, perhaps attempting to mask deficiencies and mistakes; from this perspective, faults imply a permanent lack of ability. Growth and learning opportunities are often avoided if there is a risk of failure or a revealing of weakness. A growth mindset, on the other hand, is a belief that talents and abilities can be improved and developed through learning, drive and passion. If you have a growth mindset, you are less focused on the perception of your image; instead, you tend to acknowledge your faults and seek improvements. You show a commitment to learning and are likely to pursue challenges that

[16] https://www.amazon.com/Mindset-Psychology-Carol-S-Dweck/dp/0345472322/ref=sr_1_2?crid=OA0OMYZKVQ22&dchild=1&keywords=mindset+carol+dweck&qid=1620650422&s=books&sprefix=mindset%2Cstripbooks%2C185&sr=1-2

will allow for growth opportunities. A growth mindset allows us to adapt and evolve into newer versions of our self.

A growth mindset correlates closely with other psychological principles that are essential for peak performance. For example, locus of control is an individual's belief system regarding the causes of his or her experiences and the factors to which that person attributes success or failure. This concept is usually divided into two categories: internal and external. If a person has an internal locus of control, that person attributes success to his or her own efforts and abilities. A person who expects to succeed will be more motivated and more likely to learn. A person with an external locus of control, who attributes his or her success to luck or fate, will be less likely to make the effort needed to learn. People with an external locus of control are also more likely to experience anxiety since they believe that they are not in control of their lives.

Cognitive reframing requires seeing something in a new way, in a context that allows us to recognize and appreciate positive aspects of our situation. Reframing helps us to use whatever life hands us as opportunities to be taken advantage of, rather than problems to be avoided. Breakdowns are transformed into challenges and new possibilities to experience life more fully and to become a more whole human being.

And coping refers to the human behavioral process for dealing with demands, both internal or external, in situations that are perceived as threats. Adaptive coping mechanisms help people effectively deal with their stress and might include immediate problem-solving to fix the immediate cause of the stress, benefit-finding to surface the good amidst the bad, or finding ways to turn the problem into a way to grow spiritually or emotionally.

Habit Formation

It was also Aristotle who said that "We are what we repeatedly do. Excellence, then, is not an act, but a habit." Habit is a fixed way of thinking, willing, or feeling acquired through previous repetition of a mental experience. The power of habit is that habits are automatic. The habitual action does not demand energy from your brain to make a decision. Habits are composed of a predictable loop including a cue/trigger, a routine (the action that you perform), and some reward that reinforces this action or behavior. Understanding how to build new habits (and how your current habits work) is essential for reducing cognitive load and preserving our precious cognitive resources for focus and attention.

Self-Compassion & Spirituality

Self-compassion is not antithetical to high performance. In fact, it is an essential ingredient of high performance. You can be in the midst of a stressful time or situation and persist, while at the same time telling yourself that this is indeed a hard time and being gentle with yourself. Self-compassion is grounded in three major principles:

1. Self-kindness: caring for ourselves as we would our best friends and family members
2. Recognizing our common humanity: all of us experience struggle, stress, and pain in our lives. This should connect us is a common human experience
3. Mindfulness: being present rather than denying or running from your current reality; acknowledge that this is not the best time right now but do not over exaggerate it

Spirituality is a broad concept with room for many perspectives. In general, it includes a sense of connection to something bigger than ourselves, and it typically involves a search for meaning in life. As such, it is a universal human experience—something that touches us all. Some seek spirituality through organized religious practice, so religion is a path to spirituality, but not necessarily the same thing. Books, podcasts, and lectures that discuss the larger existential themes that arise in medicine such as death and dying can help you connect with your spiritual side. Connecting to nature, finding solitude, and giving to others are ways to maintain perspective and feel grounded.

These 4 Principles for High Performing Providers should be an integral component of any professional development plan for physicians and other health care providers. They arm the individual the proper skills and practices to navigate the increasing complexity and stress in today's workplace. However, in order to properly manage and ideally prevent provider burnout, these 4 Principles must be combined with efforts to create culture and systems change in the modern health care environment.

Culture & Systems Change

Burnout is a systems issue that demands a systems-level strategy [39, 40]. To date, most health care systems have operated under the erroneous assumption that burnout is a personal issue and professional satisfaction is the responsibility of the individual. Given its impact on patient care and the bottom line—not to mention health care human capital, of course—health care organizations should have a vested interest in combatting burnout. An engaged workforce is essential for achieving institutional objectives. Unfortunately, most solutions to date have targeted the individual clinician with exercise classes and relaxation techniques, snacks and social hours for decompressing, and ways to increase efficiency and maximize productivity. There is scant evidence that these measures have had a meaningful impact [41].

Currently, there is fundamental misalignment between caregiver values and those of the healthcare system in which they operate. We do not need more resilient providers; we need more resilient systems. Organizational resilience refers to the ability of an organization to anticipate, prepare for, respond and adapt to incremental change and sudden disruptions in order to survive and prosper. And it is abundantly clear that all organizations and sectors need to be prepared for high levels of ambiguity, volatility, and complexity.

Overall, organizational science suggests that resilient organizations do not restrict resources when dealing with threats to their existence [42]. And data shows equal or greater effectiveness of organizational solutions to reduce burnout and promote well-being relative to individual-focused solutions such as those oriented around personal resilience [22, 41].

However, if we wait for get financial and emotional buy-in from medical school deans, residency program directors, clinical department chairs, and hospital executives to enable the 4 Principles for High Performing Providers, we are underappreciating our own power to make positive and productive change within our own lives and those of our colleagues. When we repeatedly feel a loss of control in a situation, it is human nature to assume a victim mentality, act in a powerless manner, and overlook opportunities for relief and change. This so-called "learned helplessness" is strongly correlated with depression and is highly prevalent in hierarchical systems. Most disturbingly, learned helplessness is a self-fulfilling prophecy.

While we must not assume the sole responsibility for creating change, nor should we underestimate our ability to play a pivotal role in the solution. Indeed, both authors of this chapter have reclaimed a locus of control by working on solutions to provider burnout. Below, we discuss ideas and opportunities to help others contribute to team culture and organizational systems change in their workplace, and in doing so, perhaps rediscover engagement [43] and renewed purpose in their work.

Team Culture Change

The ability of the team to deliver care depends on the culture and efficiency of the team. Efforts to improve both team structure and function are critical for individual and team well-being. This process includes attending to connectedness or belonging, creating psychological safety, and having team leaders with the skills to create and foster both.

Part of intrinsic motivation as defined by self-determination theory is connectedness. Feeling a sense of belonging is critical to well-being. Studies have shown that experiencing microaggressions in the workplace increases not only burn out but suicide ideation and depression as well [44]. Developing a sense of belonging for a team can be done. Psychological safety is a critical aspect to individual teams and can be cultivated by knowing individual team members. Spending time with the same team allows this individual knowledge to be developed. Also, equipping each member with the skills they need to support one another when microaggressions or other inappropriate behavior occurs is critical. Many institutions are developing upstander training to give teams this skill [45]. Finally, several institutions are allowing teams to debrief and discuss their shared experience together. Examples include Mayo's COMPASS groups where teams went out to share a meal together, which has resulted in an increase in engagement and work satisfaction [46]. We are communal creatures who thrive in an environment of acceptance and belonging. Enhancing this aspect of care team delivery adds a dimension of meaning to our workday that might otherwise not be present.

For leaders of individual teams to be effective at creating the aforementioned culture, skill sets are necessary. We can cultivate this via leadership training or leadership coaching. There are many leadership training opportunities to focus on how to create an inclusive climate and the role that leaders have in creating a team where psychological safety exists. Physicians often take a leadership role within their team, and they must know how to create high functioning and high-performing teams. Psychological safety can be measured [47] and is demonstrated when individuals are comfortable expressing and being themselves as well as sharing concerns, mistakes and discomfort without fear of embarrassment, shame, ridicule, retribution. Medicine is a classically hierarchical culture which can make psychological safety difficult to cultivate. Even something as simple as telling stories that show vulnerability and a time when you were unsure helps build their psychological safety.

Organizational Systems Change

We remain products of our environment. And today's health care environment renders execution of the 4 Principles for High Performing Providers herculean at best, impossible at worst. Any health care organization that wants to deliver high quality health care must design work processes and create an environment that fosters intrinsic motivation, achieves flow, minimizes cognitive load, supports "deep work"[17] and sustains the energy of a high performing provider workforce. Each of us, no matter our title or experience level, can use principles of design thinking to facilitate the 4 principles for our teams and colleagues.

Design Thinking

Design thinking is a collaborative problem-solving methodology used to generate human-centered solutions that are innovative, resilient and sustainable. There are five main steps to the design thinking approach which include:

1. Research and develop empathy: Take time to understand the status quo including both quantitative and qualitative data. Understand the current "user" experience from beginning to end and identify with their emotions. What are their current pain points?
2. Define the problem: Using what you learned in the research stage, identify clear problems and identify the current constraints such as limitations of time, resources & budget, and skills.
3. Ideate solutions: use visualization techniques to make complex and perhaps abstract problems more tangible. Techniques to bring possible solutions to life include mind mapping and concept sketching.

[17] https://www.calnewport.com/books/deep-work/

4. Prototype rapidly: This is a challenge for many large, bureaucratic organizations like hospitals and large provider systems where collaborative work is challenged by siloed structures and the burden of pilot data is excessive. While academic rigor is essential for clinical trials, a more experimental and iterative approach is critical to discover the ideal solutions for workplace redesign. While understandably foreign to clinician scientists, the mindset of failing fast and failing often is adaptive for prototyping and refining solutions.
5. Test your prototype with users: See if your solution resonates and works for a sample group of users. Gather feedback. Learn how to improve the prototype. Iterate and repeat.

Design Thinking for the Workplace

Design thinking methodology can help to create new workspaces that encourage relatedness, foster community, restore energy, and mitigate stress. Health care professionals confront unique challenges and encounter experiences that are distinct from other disciplines and contribute to a strong professional identity. Yet the busyness, reliance on technology, and geographic dispersion of today's physician workforce contributes to feelings of disconnectedness and isolation. Increasing productivity expectations, documentation requirements, and clerical burden are all eroding the sense of professional camaraderie that brings meaning to the intense work of patient care. In order stimulate peer support and collaboration at work, it is essential to design spaces that foster interpersonal connection.

The physician lounge, once present in nearly every hospital as a space for doctors to gather during long workdays, is now a relic of the past. The term lounge, which signifies luxury and exclusivity, for only physicians, one of many important members of growing health care teams, is an antiquated idea that conflicts with the collaborative and interdisciplinary work of modern healthcare. That said, intentionally creating time and space for connection in the workplace can help not only spur collaboration and innovation but boost camaraderie and morale. A February 2016 report[18] that grew out of the meeting of a group of consultants, physicians and other health professionals recommended that health care organizations "redesign the physical environment" to help "restore humanity" to health care. Those organizations that have reinstated a modern-day version of the physician lounge share tremendous results from what is a seemingly simple intervention.[19] A sense of connectedness is a fundamental human need. The design of modern health care workspaces can and should facilitate these connections.

As we train for health care professionals for peak performance, the workplace environment must support and facilitate the execution of such behaviors. The health care workforce must have access to nap pods and call rooms to rest and recharge during long shifts, ample superfoods and energizing snacks to avoid dips in energy,

[18] https://cdn2.hubspot.net/hubfs/506577/HealingBringsMeJoy_Final_Print_secure.pdf?t=1465835008527

[19] https://www.ama-assn.org/practice-management/physician-health/once-endangered-doctors-lounge-revived-battle-burnout

spaces for movement and standing desks to stay alert and engaged, and spaces for quiet contemplation and reflection to ease stress. Biophilic design is a concept within the building industry to increase occupant connectivity to the natural environment, which is essential for human health, productivity, and overall wellbeing. Since today's "natural habitat" is largely the built environment, biophilic design seeks to infuse nature into modern buildings and cities. There is overwhelming research that specific design elements create greater patient experience, reduce stress and enhance recovery. When patient rooms have views of nature, postoperative stays are generally shorter, less pain medication is dispensed, and overall condition improves.[20] While studies relating to healthcare staff are limited, it is clear that this population is important when making design considerations [48]. An outdoor garden may very well have positive effects on worker absences, turnover rates, work-related stress, and overall job satisfaction. Those time-tested remedies—rest, nourishment, stress relief, movement, and connection—not only heal patients, but also help bolster their caregivers.

Design Thinking as Organizational Culture

Organizations who use design thinking methodology soon discover that what perhaps begins as a process soon becomes a culture. Design thinking is a mindset and a way of working. Core organizations values like humility and integrity are necessary ingredients. In order to build organizational resilience and unlock an organizations full potential, design principles must be baked into its core philosophy and culture.

A design thinking culture could be a powerful antidote to burnout by creating a culture of cross-functional collaboration to meet the demand of the modern workplace, which require teamwork, creativity, flexibility, and critical thinking. Design thinking cultivates expansive and uninhibited ideation by embracing risk, encouraging curiosity, and brings enjoyment to the problem-solving process. Design thinking also recognizes failure as a necessary step for growth rather than focusing maniacally on efficiencies and mechanical processes that create a competitive culture and defensive workforce. Ultimately, the design thinking process and mindset breaks down the siloed, hierarchical, and bureaucratic mentality that currently typifies many health care organizations and pollutes workplace culture.

Conclusion

Performance Psychology supports the values listed above, relying on nourishing and cultivating high intrinsic motivation, optimizing environmental conditions for peak performance, and attending to and protecting high value resources. With a focus on performance, our systems will be built with the end goal of offering our

[20] https://mcdmag.com/2018/04/natures-cure-how-biophilic-design-can-enhance-healing/#.YJPryhRKgq0

patients the best experience possible. When done well, the provider offering this experience does so with a high degree of satisfaction, meaning, and purpose.

The current environment of both medical training and medical practice are not built to foster Peak performance. There is considerable effort going on both on the individual level as well as the institutional level to address issues such as burn out. It will be critical moving forward for these efforts to focus on the key principles fostering intrinsic motivation, attending to the science of attention, looking at time as an unrenewable and precious asset, and focusing on peak performance. The focus on these four key principles can be done in the current structure of process improvement or with a lens towards design thinking. There is much we can learn from other industries and how to improve our focus on these key principles in order to create an environment optimal for learning and patient care delivery but it's sustainable for long-term engagement.

Resources/References

1. Mata DA, Ramos MA, Bansal N, Khan R, Guille C, Di Angelantonio E, Sen S. Prevalence of depression and depressive symptoms among resident physicians: a systematic review and meta-analysis. JAMA. 2015;314:2373–83. https://doi.org/10.1001/jama.2015.15845.
2. Rotenstein LS, Ramos MA, Torre M, Segal JB, Peluso MJ, Guille C, Sen S, Mata DA. Prevalence of depression, depressive symptoms, and suicidal ideation among medical students. JAMA. 2016;316:2214–36. https://doi.org/10.1001/jama.2016.17324.
3. Shanafelt T, Gorringe G, Menaker R, et al. Impact of organizational leadership on physician burnout and satisfaction. Mayo Clin Proc. 2015;90(4):432–40.
4. Maslach C, Jackson SE, Leiter MP. Maslach burnout inventory manual. 4th ed. Mind Garden Inc: Menlo Park; 2016.
5. Maslach C, Leiter MP. The truth about burnout: how organizations cause personal stress and what to do about it. San Francisco: Jossey-Bass; 1997.
6. Center C, Davis M, Detre T, Ford DE, Hansbrough W, Hendin H, Laszlo J, Litts DA, Mann J, Mansky PA, Michels R, Miles SH, Proujansky R, Reynolds CF, Silverman MM. Confronting depression and suicide in physicians: a consensus statement. JAMA. 2003;289:3161–6.
7. Oreskovich MR, Kaups KL, Balch CM, Hanks JB, Satele D, Sloan J, Meredith C, Buhl A, Dyrbye LN, Shanafelt TD. The prevalence of alcohol use disorders among American surgeons. Arch Surg. 2012;147:168–74.
8. Mata DA, Ramos MA, Bansal N, et al. Prevalence of depression and depressive symptoms among resident physicians: a systematic review and meta-analysis. JAMA. 2015;314(22):2373–83. https://doi.org/10.1001/jama.2015.15845.
9. Shanafelt TD, Balch CM, Dyrbye LN, Bechamps G, Russell T, Satele D, Rummans T, Swartz K, Novotny PJ, Sloan J, Oreskovich MR. Suicidal ideation among American surgeons. Arch Surg. 2011;146:54–62.
10. Schernhammer E. Taking their own lives – the high rate of physician suicide. N Engl J Med. 2005;352(24):2473–6.
11. Panagioti M, Geraghty K, Johnson J, et al. Association between physician burnout and patient safety, professionalism, and patient satisfaction: a systematic review and meta-analysis. JAMA Intern Med. 2018;178:1317–30.
12. Shanafelt TD, Balch CM, Bechamps GJ, Russell T, Dyrbye L, Satele D, Collicott P, Novotny PJ, Sloan J, Freischlag JA. Burnout and career satisfaction among American surgeons. Ann Surg. 2009;250:463–71. https://doi.org/10.1097/SLA.0b013e3181ac4dfd.

13. Shanafelt TD, Sloan J, Satele D, Balch C. Why do surgeons consider leaving practice? J Am Coll Surg. 2010;212:421–2.
14. Halbesleben JRB, Rathert C. Linking physician burnout and patient outcomes: exploring the dyadic relationship between physicians and patients. Health Care Manag Rev. 2008;33:29–39.
15. Shanafelt TD, Balch CM, Bechamps G, Russell T, Dyrbye L, Satele D, Collicott P, Novotny PJ, Sloan J, Freischlag J. Burnout and medical errors among American surgeons. Ann Surg. 2010;251:995–1000. https://doi.org/10.1097/SLA.0b013e3181bfdab3.
16. Han S, Shanafelt TD, Sinsky CA, Awad KM, Dyrbye LN, Fiscus LC, Trockel M, Goh J. Estimating the attributable cost of physician burnout in the United States. Ann Intern Med. 2019;170(11):784–90. https://doi.org/10.7326/M18-1422. Epub 2019 May 28. PMID: 31132791.
17. Fibuch E, Ahmed A. Physician turnover: a costly problem. Physician Leadersh J. 2015;2:22–5.
18. Buchbinder SB, Wilson M, Melick CF, Powe NR. Estimates of costs of primary care physician turnover. Am J Manag Care. 1999;5:1431–8.
19. Physician burnout is a public health crisis: a message to our fellow health care CEOs. Health Affairs Blog. March 28, 2017.
20. Krasner MS, Epstein RM, Beckman H, Suchman AL, Chapman B, Mooney CJ, Quill TE. Association of an educational program in mindful communication with burnout, empathy, and attitudes among primary care physicians. JAMA. 2009;302:1284–93.
21. Dunn PM, Arnetz BB, Christensen JF, Homer L. Meeting the imperative to improve physician well-being: assessment of an innovative program. J Gen Intern Med. 2007;22:1544–52.
22. West CP, Dyrbye LN, Erwin PJ, Shanafelt TD. Interventions to prevent and reduce physician burnout: a systematic review and meta-analysis. Lancet. 2016;388(10057):2272–81. https://doi.org/10.1016/S0140-6736(16)31279-X. Epub 2016 Sep 28. PMID: 27692469.
23. Panagioti M, Panagopoulou E, Bower P, Lewith G, Kontopantelis E, Chew-Graham C, Dawson S, van Marwijk H, Geraghty K, Esmail A. Controlled interventions to reduce burnout in physicians: a systematic review and meta-analysis. JAMA Intern Med. 2017;177(2):195–205. https://doi.org/10.1001/jamainternmed.2016.7674. PMID: 27918798.
24. Anon. Factors affecting clinician well-being and resilience – conceptual model – clinician well-being knowledge hub. 2021. Retrieved April 26, 2021. https://nam.edu/clinicianwellbeing/resources/factors-affecting-clinician-well-being-and-resilience-conceptual-model/.
25. Shanafelt TD, Noseworthy JH. Executive leadership and physician well-being: nine organizational strategies to promote engagement and reduce burnout. Mayo Clin Proc. 2016;92(1):129–46.
26. Basil MD. Multiple Resource Theory. In: Seel N.M. (eds) Encyclopedia of the Sciences of Learning. Springer, Boston, MA. 2012:2384–85.
27. Baddeley A. Working memory, thought, and action. Oxford: New York Oxford University Press; 2005.
28. Sweller J. Cognitive Load Theory. In: Seel N.M. (eds) Encyclopedia of the Sciences of Learning. Springer, Boston, MA. 2012:601–5.
29. Bourne LE, Yaroush RA. Stress and cognition: a cognitive psychological perspective. 2001.
30. Leahy W, Sweller J. Cognitive load theory, resource depletion and the delayed testing effect. Educ Psychol Rev. 2019;31(2):457–78.
31. Harry E, Sinsky C, Dyrbye LN, Makowski MS, et al. Physician task load and the risk of burnout among US physicians in a national survey. Jt Comm J Qual Patient Saf. 2021;47(2):76–85.
32. Kissler MJ, Kissler K, Burden M. Toward a medical ecology of attention. N Engl J Med. 2021;384(4):299–301.
33. Anon. Journal of Experimental Psychology: Human Perception and Performance | APA. 2021. Retrieved April 26, 2021. https://www.apa.org/pubs/journals/xhp/.
34. Kumaraiah D, Yip N, Ivascu N, Hill L. Innovative ICU physician care models: COVID-19 pandemic at NewYork-Presbyterian. NEJM Catal Innov Care Deliv. 2020;1(2).
35. Stajduhar T. Jackson Physician Search, 2021. On the verge of a physician turnover epidemic. Physician retention survey results — February 2021.

36. Ajao A, Nystrom SV, Koonin LM, Patel A, Howell DR, Baccam P, Lant T, Malatino E, Chamberlin M, Meltzer MI. Assessing the capacity of the US health care system to use additional mechanical ventilators during a large-scale public health emergency. Disaster Med Public Health Prep. 2015;9(6):634–41.
37. Reivich KJ, Seligman ME, McBride S. Master resilience training in the U.S. Army. Am Psychol. 2011;66(1):25–34. https://doi.org/10.1037/a0021897.
38. Griffith J, West C. Master resilience training and its relationship to individual well-being and stress buffering among army national guard soldiers. J Behav Health Serv Res. 2013;40(2):140–55. https://doi.org/10.1007/s11414-013-9320-8.
39. Williams ES, Konrad TR, Linzer M, et al. Physician, practice, and patient characteristics related to primary care physician physical and mental health: results from the Physician Worklife Study. Health Serv Res. 2002;37(1):121–43.
40. Bodenheimer T, Sinsky C. From triple to quadruple aim: care of the patient requires care of the provider. Ann Fam Med. 2014;12(6):573–6.
41. Panagioti M, Panagopoulou E, Bower P, et al. Controlled interventions to reduce burnout in physicians: a systematic review and meta-analysis. JAMA Intern Med. 2017;177(2):195–205.
42. Gittell JH, Cameron K, Lim S, Rivas V. Relationships, layoffs, and organizational resilience: airline industry responses to September 11. J Appl Behav Sci. 2006;42:300–29.
43. Shimazu A, Schaufeli WB. Work engagement: an emerging concept in occupational health psychology. Biosci Trends. 2008;2(1):2.
44. Hu Y-Y, Ellis R, Hewitt D, Yang A, Cheung E, Moskowitz J, et al. Discrimination, abuse, harassment, and burnout in surgical residency training. N Engl J Med. 2019; https://doi.org/10.1056/NEJMsa1903759.
45. Evans M, Rosenbaum L, Malina D, Morrissey S, Rubin E. Diagnosing and treating systemic racism. N Engl J Med. 2020; https://doi.org/10.1056/NEJMe2021693.
46. Mahmoud NN, Rothenberger D. From burnout to well-being: a focus on resilience. Clin Colon Rectal Surg. 2019; https://doi.org/10.1055/s-0039-1692710.
47. Edmondson A. Psychological safety and learning behavior in work teams. Adm Sci Q. 1999; https://doi.org/10.2307/2666999.
48. Huisman E, Morales E, Hoof JV, Kort H. Healing environment: a review of the impact of physical environmental factors on users. Build Environ. 2012;58:70–80. https://doi.org/10.1016/j.buildenv.2012.06.016.

Helpful Resources

https://www.ahrq.gov/prevention/clinician/ahrq-works/burnout/index.html.
https://www.medscape.com/slideshow/2020-lifestyle-burnout-6012460.
https://nam.edu/burnout-among-health-care-professionals-a-call-to-explore-and-address-this-underrecognized-threat-to-safe-high-quality-care/.
https://nam.edu/systems-approaches-to-improve-patient-care-by-supporting-clinician-well-being/.
https://cdn2.hubspot.net/hubfs/506577/HealingBringsMeJoy_Final_Print_secure.pdf?t=1465835008527.

9 Financial Considerations for the Healthcare Professional

James M. Dahle

While not every doctor enjoyed medical school, I consider it to be four of the best years of my life. I enjoyed the camaraderie and fascinating material, but most of all I loved applying that knowledge in an effort to help other people. Likewise, residency was my favorite job that I ever had. Do not get me wrong, the hours were long and I certainly would not volunteer to do it again, but I found it very fulfilling to be making a real difference while becoming more and more competent each week. I can remember thinking I would be willing to practice medicine even if it only paid $30,000 a year.

Apparently, most of my peers do not feel the same way. I did a recent survey of hundreds of doctors. It was just a Twitter poll, not some scientific survey, but I asked doctors how much they would work if they had enough money to never need to work again. You might be surprised by their answers:

- 35% said they would quit practicing completely
- 55% said they would cut back on how much they are practicing
- 10% said they would continue to practice as much as they currently do

Yes, that is right. 90% of physicians are practicing either partially or completely for the money. I suppose that is not all that different from most other people in the world, but for some reason, healthcare professionals see ourselves as being different and dedicated to a higher cause. Over the years I have met thousands of burned out doctors who want nothing more than to cut back on how much they practice or leave medicine completely. I find it very difficult to reconcile the presence, attitudes, and desires of those doctors with the excitement I see in pre-meds who have just received their first acceptance to medical school or fourth year medical students who just matched into their chosen specialty.

J. M. Dahle (✉)
Department of Emergency Medicine, Jordan Valley Medical Center, West Jordan, UT, USA
e-mail: Editor@whitecoatinvestor.com

© The Author(s), under exclusive license to Springer Nature Switzerland AG 2022

P. K. Louie et al. (eds.), *The Successful Health Care Professional's Guide*,
https://doi.org/10.1007/978-3-030-95950-0_9

I am now a mid-career emergency physician. Thanks to good planning and some fortunate events in my life, I am now financially independent, meaning I do not need the money I earn practicing medicine and in fact give more than I earn practicing to charity each year. From a financial perspective, medicine has essentially turned into a well-paying hobby for me. Nobody really knows for sure if they would practice medicine for little or no compensation until they are financially independent.

Financial independence has allowed me to practice on my terms. I can practice when, where, and how much I want. My recommendations to patients can be completely pure, since it makes no difference at all to me how much I get paid for treating them. I feel zero pressure from metric-driven administrators to do anything that might result in poor patient care. What are they going to do, fire me? Now that I am financially independent, being fired would have zero impact on my financial life. Perhaps it would impact the local charities a bit, but that would be the only financial effect. Now you can see why getting your financial ducks in a row can reduce burnout and allow you to be a better family member, person, and doctor.

If you are like those who have come before you (and you almost surely are) chances are very good (90% apparently) that within 10 years of finishing your education and training that you will want to practice medicine less than full time or perhaps not at all. The ability to do this is entirely within your grasp. If you will acquire a relatively small body of knowledge and a relatively small amount of discipline, and apply both of them to your financial life, you can also find yourself in a position similar to mine at mid-career. Even if you decide that you really are the person you told the medical school admissions committee you were in your essay and see full-time medicine as a calling more than a job, financial independence will still allow you to be even more dedicated to your patients.

In this chapter, I will outline the pathway to early financial independence.

Personal finance is both personal and finance. When I say personal, I mean it depends a great deal on your values, goals, and behavior. When I say finance, I am talking about math and technical knowledge. To be honest, personal finance is 80% behavioral and only 20% finance. While you will need to be able to do fourth grade math and learn some new terminology, the primary determinant of your success will be what you do, not what you know.

Recognize that you will also need to personalize the information you read in this chapter. Your situation is different in some small way from everybody else's situation. You have certain advantages and disadvantages that others do not. Perhaps you will wish to be more or less aggressive in reaching financial independence. That is all perfectly fine. I simply want you to be aware of the tools and knowledge required to get there. It is up to you what you do with them.

Perhaps the first concept to discuss is the difference between income and wealth. Society, including government agencies such as the IRS, routinely confuse these two concepts. Income is how much money you make each year. Wealth is how much money you have left at the end of the year. Although we think of a rich person as having a lot of stuff and spending a lot of money, in reality, wealth is exactly the opposite. Wealth is what you do not see. Wealth is money that was earned but not spent. Millionaires become millionaires precisely because they did not spend a million dollars that they could have spent.

As a health care professional of just about any type, your greatest wealth-building tool is your income. Perhaps you own a practice, have a bit of an entrepreneurial streak, or received a significant inheritance. But if you are like most docs, you are a first-generation physician, paid for your schooling primarily with student loans, and will spend most of your career as an employee. If you ever want to build wealth (and you will need to if you want to be financially independent), that wealth will have to be carved out of your income.

You might be surprised to learn that there are doctors who are living hand to mouth on $300,000 or even $400,000 a year. If you do not think you can blow through that much money in a year, let me demonstrate how it is done for a family of four.

- Income: $300,000
  - Federal incomes taxes: $75,455
  - FICA (payroll) taxes: $13,787
  - State taxes (CA): $24,589
  - Health insurance (your share): $9000
- Take home pay: $177,169
  - Mortgage: $45,000
  - Property taxes: $5000
  - Homeowner's insurance: $1000
  - Student loan payments: $34,000
  - Private school tuition (2 kids): $30,000
  - Disability insurance: $6000
  - Term life insurance: $2000
  - Utilities, cell phone, internet: $8000
  - Car payments: $12,000
  - Auto insurance: $1000
  - Total Fixed Expenses: $144,000
- Amount left after fixed expenses: $33,169
  - Groceries: $12,000
  - Eating out: $4000
  - Clothing: $2000
  - Gasoline: $6000
  - Children's' activities: $2000
  - Vacations: $5000
  - Entertainment: $2169
  - Total variable expenses: $33,169
- Amount left after variable expenses: $0

See what I mean? Hand to mouth. Do you see what is not in this budget? There are no "extra" student loan payments, just the required ones. No extra car payments or mortgage payments either. There is no saving up for a boat, a second home, or even a car. There is no saving for college, no saving for retirement, and certainly no helping out of family members or donating to charities. There is not a single expense in this budget that a typical attending physician would find outrageous, but when you put it all together, it is obvious that this family will never build any wealth. Guess what? There are a lot of doctor families that live just like this.

The Medscape Physician Wealth and Debt Report 2016 [1] was a survey of doctors asking about their wealth and debt levels. In my opinion, the most important question in that survey was when the doctors were asked about their net worth. Net worth is the measurement of wealth; it is everything you own minus everything you owe. Medscape then stratified the results by age. While doctors in their 30s were generally quite poor, you might be surprised to learn that a lot of doctors in their 60s were also quite poor. Approximately 12% of doctors in their 60s had a net worth of less than $500,000. That's everything—bank accounts, retirement accounts, investments, home equity, cars, clothing, furniture, boats, you name it. 25% of doctors in their 60s had less than $1 million in net worth. These doctors had earned a six-figure income for decades and had very little of it left.

How does that happen? Mostly it occurs simply because the doctors spent everything they made. Medscape does this survey every year and the results are not getting much better. Unfortunately, they stopped breaking out the data by age like they did in 2016. But even in 2020, 57% of doctors admitted they were living hand to mouth or worse [2].

I want you to resolve right now that you will not let this happen to you. You can avoid this financial catastrophe simply by deciding you will not spend your entire income. You will actually carve something out of a top 1–2% income and use it to build wealth.

Becoming rich (use wealthy, comfortable, or financially independent if you prefer those terms) is not particularly complicated. There are four steps:

1. Earn a lot of money
2. Do not spend a lot of money
3. Invest the difference in some reasonable way
4. Ensure you do not lose your money to death, disability, divorce, or dirt bags.

It really is that simple. As a physician, dentist, advanced practice clinician, physical therapist, optometrist or other high income professional, you already earn a lot of money compared to most people. You have already done the hard part. Now you just need to complete the last three steps and you will eventually be wealthy.

Remember that the median American retiree only has a net worth of about a quarter million dollars, less than you might make in a single year [3]. If your goal is to just be in the top half, you can probably get there just from paying off your mortgage. However, I would encourage you to set your sights a little higher.

So how much should you save? In order to retire comfortably (i.e. maintain your standard of living in retirement) in their 60s, a typical worker needs to save about 15% of their gross income just for retirement throughout their career. Physicians, due to their late start, higher tax burden, and lower relative Social Security benefits, need to save a little more, perhaps 20% of gross income. If they wish to retire early, they will need to save even more. In fact, the FIRE (Financial Independence, Retire Early) community has shown that when you can retire depends primarily on your savings rate. Extreme savings rates (50%+ of gross income) can allow for retirement in less than a decade. The flip side is also true; if you save 5% or less of your gross income, you will become eligible for Social Security before you become financially independent.

Perhaps the most significant financial obstacle for a young doctor, whether in training or the first few years out of training, is dealing with a massive student loan burden. Approximately ¾ of doctors pay for their schooling primarily with student loans. The other quarter is divided between those whose family paid for their education and those paying for schooling with contracts such as those available from the military, National Health Service Corps, or an MD/PhD program. The cost of education has skyrocketed, particularly for graduate programs such as medicine. The median debt burden for MDs is now over $200,000, and that number is already over $250,000 and rising rapidly for DOs and dentists. If a graduate combines the median debt burden with the median physician income (currently in the neighborhood of $275,000 as this chapter is written), everything can work out just fine. Going to medical school is still a good investment.

However, if someone combines a lowest quartile doctor income with a highest quartile student loan burden, things do not work out nearly as well. It simply is not a good financial move to borrow $600,000 to get a job that pays only $150,000. As Dave Ramsey has famously said, "You don't get a pass on math" just because you have dreams and want to do something good in the world. Run the numbers early so you have an idea of what you are going to owe by the time you are done training. Then make sure your career plan will allow you to deal with the consequences of your decisions to go to professional school and pay for it with student loans.

There are three main ways that doctors deal with their student loan burden. The most commonly used method is to pay the loans back. This is the only option available on private student loans, but also still one of the best for dealing with federal loans. The other two options are only available with federal loans—tax-free Public Service Loan Forgiveness and fully taxable Income Driven Repayment Plan Forgiveness. We will discuss each of these in turn.

Paying off your student loans is very straightforward, even if it is not necessarily easy. You simply take the difference between what you earn and what you live on and direct some or all of that money toward your student loans. You can also refinance the loans to a lower rate. Great deals on student loan refinancing can be found at https://www.whitecoatinvestor.com. You can get the best rates available plus several hundred dollars cash back each time you refinance by going through the links on that site. The lower your interest rate, the more of your payments that go toward principal instead of interest.

Financially savvy doctors have discovered that if they will live like a resident for a few years after completing their training that they can pay off their student loans within 5 years of residency completion. The numbers are very straightforward. Imagine you earn the median physician income of $275,000. Perhaps you are paying $90,000 in tax. That leaves $185,000. If you live on $60,000, a typical resident salary and the median American household income, that leaves $125,000 with which to pay off student loans. At that rate, you can pay off $250,000 in student loans in just over 2 years and $500,000 in student loans in just over 4 years. Even if these doctors are also maximizing contributions to their retirement accounts and saving up a down payment for their dream home, most of those who will live like a resident will still pay off their student loans completely within 2–5 years of residency completion. The same financial muscles they built while accomplishing that goal will serve them well as they continue to save and invest toward financial independence.

Residents can refinance their private loans at any time, but they should not necessarily refinance their federal loans until they are sure that they will be going down the "pay off the student loans" pathway. Once you refinance your federal loans, you have closed the door on the other two pathways.

The second pathway is Public Service Loan Forgiveness. This is an excellent choice for somebody with a large amount of federal student loans who completed a long residency, ± a fellowship, and is working as an academic doctor. Doctors can have their remaining student loans forgiven tax-free after just 3–7 years of post-training payments. It is entirely possible for doctors in this situation to pay less than $100,000 toward a $400,000+ student loan burden and still be rid of it within just a few years of residency completion. However, there are some very specific rules involved with Public Service Loan Forgiveness, and you must comply with all of them in order to receive forgiveness. Here are the five rules:

1. You must have eligible student loans. Only direct, federal student loans are eligible. Private loans cannot be forgiven.
2. You must be enrolled in an eligible repayment program. Most borrowers are enrolled in an Income Driven Repayment (IDR) program such as Income Based Repayment (IBR), Pay As You Earn (PAYE) or Revised Pay As You Earn (REPAYE), but there are some other options.
3. You must be an employee of a non-profit, sometimes called a 501(c)3, or a governmental agency. This includes most academic, VA, and military positions.
4. You must work full-time.
5. You must make 120 on-time, monthly payments. They do not need to be consecutive, but there must be 120 of them.

Basically, if you make payments for 10 years while working for a non-profit (which includes most residency and fellowship programs), anything else you owe is forgiven tax-free. Be sure to fill out the annual certification forms and the forgiveness application itself correctly and keep careful records of every one of those 120 payments. Loan servicing companies tend to do a poor job of counting to 120.

The third pathway, IDR forgiveness, is less ideal than the above two for most physicians and advanced practice clinicians, but it can make a lot of sense for a select few with a very high debt to income ratio of 1.5–2 or higher. It is a much better pathway for other professionals who generally have a higher debt to income ratio such as veterinarians, optometrists, many attorneys, and pharmacists.

If you have a very high debt to income ratio, but are not willing or able to work for a PSLF-qualifying employer, then look into IDR forgiveness. Each of the IDR programs has a forgiveness aspect to it. While "the deal" is nowhere near as good as PSLF, the work requirements for IDR forgiveness are much more lenient.

Instead of only making payments for 10 years, you will need to make payments for 20–25 years. Instead of receiving tax-free forgiveness, with an IDR forgiveness program the amount forgiven will be added to your taxable income for the year you receive forgiveness. This will result in a massive "tax bomb" that you had better be prepared to pay. If you thought it was bad to owe money to the Department of Education, wait until you owe it to the Department of the Treasury (i.e. the Internal Revenue Service.) So those who go down this pathway not only need to make their required payments, but they also need to save and invest thousands of dollars every year toward that tax bomb. Obviously if you can qualify for PSLF, go for PSLF, not IDR forgiveness. PSLF is so much better that it is likely you will come out ahead taking a PSLF-qualifying job even if it pays less, treats you worse, and/or requires you to move across the country for a few years.

The benefit of IDR forgiveness over PSLF is that you do not have to work for a non-profit or a governmental agency. You can work for anyone you like, or nobody at all. There is no work requirement. Since the payments are all income based, if you have little to no income, the payments are very small or even $0. However, if you have a typical physician income and a typical physician student loan debt burden, you will pay off your student loans before being eligible for IDR forgiveness. A single doctor enrolled in PAYE with an income of $275,000 who owes $205,000 in student loans at 6% would be required to make payments of $2141 per month ($25,692 per year). At that rate, the loan would be paid off in 11 years. Even with a five-year residency, the loans are still paid off in16 years, 4 years before that doctor would be eligible for PAYE forgiveness. Without a high debt to income ratio, there is no IDR forgiveness. There are just many years of relatively high-interest IDR payments made to student loan servicing companies who generally offer poor service. In those situations, you are far better off just refinancing the loans, living like a resident for a few years, and paying them off.

If you need help running the numbers on your student loan situation to decide which pathway is best for your federal student loans, considering spending an hour of your time and a few hundred dollars with https://studentloanadvice.com to get professional advice. It may save you tens or even hundreds of thousands of dollars.

There is an entire chapter in this book about disability and term life insurance. I suggest you read it very carefully. Insurance is a critical aspect of financial planning. You simply cannot self-insure against several financial catastrophes in life.

Unless you are financially independent or married to someone who will support you in the event you become permanently disabled, you need to buy disability insurance. Most physicians find it is best if at least some of their disability insurance comes from a private, individual, portable, own-occupation, specialty-specific policy issued by one of the "Big 5" companies (Guardian, The Standard, Ameritas,

Mass Mutual, and Principal). You want something that is actually going to pay out if you become disabled enough that you cannot practice your specialty, even if you are able to do something else for a fraction of the pay. The most valuable asset of most young docs is their ability to turn their time into money at a very high rate. Most attending physicians buy a tax-free benefit of $10–20,000 per month. Unfortunately, it is not cheap; they tend to pay $200–1200 per month for that benefit.

If you have dependents and are not financially independent, you probably also need a large term life policy. If you should happen to die, the death benefit of the policy replaces your future income and what it would have purchased, including paying off a mortgage, funding college for your children, and supporting your spouse for the rest of your spouse's life. For a typical attending physician, that means a death benefit of $1–5 million. The good news is that life insurance is typically much cheaper than disability insurance. A $1–5 million, 20–30 year level term policy for a healthy young doctor will typically cost between $25 and $200 per month.

Beware financial salespeople who push whole life insurance on young doctors. This insurance provides a death benefit throughout your whole life, not just for a 20- or 30-year term. However, since everyone will eventually die, this benefit costs much more than term life insurance, sometimes ten times as much or more. It is not a good way to provide a death benefit during your working years, and despite how hard that agent works to sell it to you, it is rarely the best way to pay for anything else in your life either. If you need help procuring disability or term life insurance from an expert who will not also try to sell you whole life insurance, check out the recommended list of agents at https://www.whitecoatinvestor.com.

Becoming seriously ill or injured is also a financial catastrophe that is folly to try to self-insure. If your employer does not provide it, be sure to purchase health insurance yourself. It is even more expensive than disability insurance, but there is a reason for that—it gets used! Take a look at the bills sent out in your name sometime. I assure you it is far better to be on the sending end of those bills than the receiving end, especially when you do not have health insurance. Many doctors who find themselves purchasing health insurance on the open market are surprised to learn that it may cost $10,000–25,000 per year to insure a family. They had no idea that their employers had been picking up the lion's share of that tab for them for years.

Professional liability insurance also addresses a serious financial catastrophe. On average, physicians are sued about once a career. Some specialties are higher risk than others, such as neurosurgery, obstetrics, and general surgery. It would not be unusual at all for you to acquire a six-figure judgment at some point in your career. This is worth insuring against. Not only does a malpractice insurance policy pay for any settlements or court-mandated judgments, but it also pays for your defense. The cost of malpractice insurance has trended down over the last couple of decades, but still usually costs thousands to tens of thousands per year even for just a million dollars in coverage. Make sure you carry as much coverage as most other docs in your specialty and geographic area. Occurrence coverage is more valuable than claims-made coverage, since it will cover events that occurred during the time period the policy was in place, whether the claim was made during that period or not. If you have claims-made coverage, you (or your previous or next employer) should purchase a "tail" insurance policy against the possibility of later claims.

You probably also want to insure your valuable property, such as your home, real estate investments, automobiles, and toys such as boats. 1 out of 400 homes burns down every year, and most doctors cannot afford to replace theirs if it does.

Homeowner's, renter's, and auto insurance policies also usually contain some liability protection. While this will not protect you from malpractice liability, it does protect you from claims that may occur when your 16-year-old drives your suburban into the local CEO's BMW, when somebody slips and falls off your porch, or when someone sues you for libel. However, the amount of liability protection in many of these policies is pathetically low. Some states only require you to carry $50,000 of auto insurance despite the fact that there are plenty of cars on the road worth more than that, and that doesn't include the economic value of the occupants, their medical bills, and their future earnings. You should purchase a personal liability (or umbrella) policy that sits on top of your auto and home policy to provide additional protection. It will be much cheaper than your malpractice coverage, typically costing just a few hundred dollars a year for millions of dollars of coverage.

With a student loan and insurance plan in place, many doctors now turn to their spending and investing plans. These are two opposite sides of the same coin; the more you spend, the less you can save and invest and vice versa. Naturally, your hearse will not have a trailer hitch. It does not do you any good to be the richest doctor in the graveyard. So your goal should not necessarily be simply to acquire the most wealth possible. Your goal should be to save enough to provide for your later years while using money to improve your life, help those around you, and perhaps enjoy a few luxuries along the way.

When considering your spending plan (or budget), I would encourage you to focus on the "big rocks", rather than the "small rocks." Big rocks include taxes, your housing costs, your transportation costs, and the cost of insurance. Small rocks are things such as hobbies, eating out, and the infamous daily latte'. You'll build wealth a lot faster by living in a house that costs half as much than you will from using massive daily willpower to skip that latte'.

Buy a house when it makes sense for you to do so. That usually means a period of time when you will be in the house for at least 5 years and have a stable personal and professional life. Yes, that means most residents probably are going to come out behind when they buy a house. They simply are not in the house long enough for it to appreciate enough to overcome the substantial transaction costs of buying and selling a house (about 15% round trip.) Too many mistakenly assumed that because the mortgage cost less than rent that it was a good idea to buy.

Likewise, many Americans have over a million dollars sitting in their driveway. Consider the difference between driving a fancy, luxury car and a used economy car. Edmunds.com offers a calculator that shows you the five-year cost of ownership of a vehicle. An Audi A8 costs about $80,000 in its first 5 years, including $30,000 of depreciation. That works out to be about $16,000 per year. A Honda Civic of the same year costs about $31,000 over 5 years, or about $6200 per year. They both have four doors and will get you back and forth reliably to the hospital. Yet one costs $10,000 more per year. Starting at age 20 and going to age 65, $10,000 per year invested at 8% grows to $3.9 million! Even if you don't start until age 35, it still grows to $1.1 million. If you buy Honda Civics that are already 5–10 years old, you will save even more.

Now, I personally believe that most doctors can afford to drive a nicer car than a Honda Civic for most of their career and still retire as multi-millionaires. But if you find that you're a little behind in your retirement savings or just want to retire earlier or wealthier, take a long hard look at what is sitting in your driveway, how you're paying for it, and whether you're willing to work an extra shift or take an additional call every month in order to drive it. Imagine life without a car payment, then allow yourself to realize that I (and many people like me) have never had a car payment in our entire life. If we only had $2000 (or $5000 or $10,000) for a car, we drove a $2000 (or $5000 or $10,000) car until we had the money to buy something nicer. Basic transportation starts at $2000 and reliable transportation starts at $5000. That's a 10-year-old Civic with 120,000 miles on it. That car is only halfway through its life.

Naturally, you will want to avoid blowing your hard-earned money on interest whenever possible, especially relatively high interest rates. Credit cards are not made for credit, they are made for convenience so you can buy airline tickets online, buy gas at the pump, and avoid a few trips to the ATM. If you find you are carrying a balance on a credit card month to month, you have proven to yourself that you cannot handle credit cards safely. Cut them up and use a debit card, even if it is less convenient.

The goal is to avoid living hand to mouth. Not only do you need to live within your means, but you need to carve 20% or more of your gross income out to use to build wealth. I recommend physicians who want to retire in their 60s save 20% of their gross income just for retirement throughout their career. College is extra. A second home or Tesla is extra. Retiring early is extra.

Once you have carved a significant amount of money out of your annual budget in order to invest for your future, you will need to decide what accounts to invest it in. It turns out the government wants you to save for retirement, so they will subsidize your efforts to do so. That subsidy is called a retirement account and they come in numerous flavors, including 401(k)s, 403(b)s, 457(b)s, and Roth IRAs. In addition, your employer may also subsidize your retirement by putting money into a pension or retirement account. Sometimes that subsidy comes in the form of a "match", where the employer only puts money in the account if the employee also defers some of their salary into the account. Not getting your entire match is like leaving part of your salary on the table.

Most retirement accounts are defined contribution plans, where the eventual value of the account depends on the performance of the underlying investments. There are two main types of these accounts, tax-deferred (sometimes called traditional) and tax-free (sometimes called Roth, after Senator William Roth who sponsored the legislation that resulted in the Roth IRA.) A tax-deferred account provides a tax deduction for the year in which the contribution is made.

Withdrawals from the account in retirement are considered fully taxable income. A tax-free account provides no up-front deduction, but withdrawals are completely tax-free. Both types of accounts eliminate the "tax-drag" that occurs from the taxation of interest, dividends, and capital gains as the investments grow in value. This causes the money in retirement accounts to grow faster than it would outside retirement accounts. In addition, retirement accounts provide substantial estate planning and asset protection benefits compared to non-retirement investing accounts.

Each type of retirement account has rules about how much can be contributed, when and how money can be withdrawn, and what types of investments can be placed inside the account. It is critical that you understand the various types of these tax-advantaged accounts available to you so that you can maximize these benefits while minimizing any downsides and hassles. You will want to check with the human resources personnel of your employer to learn about any employer provided retirement accounts. They are required to give you a summary plan document for those plans, but only if you ask for it. Be sure to read the document, log in to the account, figure out what you're investing in, and make sure you're contributing enough not only to get the match (if any), but to hit the maximum account contribution.

If you are self-employed as an independent contractor, open an individual (sometimes called solo) 401(k). If you own a practice with employees, seek out competent professional assistance to determine which type of retirement plan is best for your business. We keep a list of recommended professionals at https://www.whitecoatinvestor.com.

You are also able to contribute to Individual Retirement Arrangements (IRAs). Most doctors contribute to a Roth IRA, and due to some unwieldy contribution rules, have to do it "through the backdoor" by contributing first to a traditional IRA before moving the money into a Roth IRA. Even if their spouse is not working, they can also contribute to a spousal Roth IRA by the same process.

Health Saving Accounts (HSA) can also function as a type of retirement account. In fact, they may be the most tax-advantaged accounts of all. Not only do you get an up-front tax deduction for contributions just like a tax-deferred retirement account and the tax-protected growth of all retirement accounts, but you also get tax-free withdrawals (just like a tax-free retirement account) so long as the withdrawal is used for health care. A lot of people do not realize the money in these accounts can be invested in mutual funds just like a 401(k). Unlike a Flexible Spending Account (FSA), an HSA can be rolled over year to year indefinitely.

If you are not able to fit all of your retirement savings (whether 20% of gross income or more) into retirement accounts, you will need to invest some of it outside of retirement accounts. That may mean purchasing mutual funds inside a non-qualified brokerage account (often called a taxable account) or perhaps buying real estate investment properties. While not as robust as the tax, estate, and asset protection advantages of a retirement account, investments often qualify for significant tax advantages such as lower qualified dividend tax rates, lower long-term capital gains tax rates, and the ability to use depreciation to avoid paying taxes on rental income.

Once you have decided the accounts into which you will invest your retirement money, you will next need to select the actual investments. Think of an investing account as a type of luggage—whether a suitcase, backpack, or truck, and the investments as different types of clothing—parkas, dresses, or swimsuits. Any type of investment can go into any type of account just like any type of clothing can go into any type of luggage.

The overall performance of your portfolio (mixture of investments) mostly depends on the ratio of the various types of investments in the account, such as stocks, bonds, and real estate. Savvy investors decide on an overall strategy for the portfolio before selecting investments. For example, my own portfolio is 60% stocks, 20% bonds, and 20% real estate. If real estate has a particularly good year, I put less money into real estate and more money into stocks and bonds and vice versa. This allows me to hold the risk in my portfolio constant. Over time, every type of investment (asset class) will have its day in the sun, and I want to own it when it does. A diversified portfolio holds multiple asset classes. Naturally, a diversified portfolio always holds something that is not doing particularly well at the time. Diversification works, even when you do not want it to!

If you need help deciding on your investment plan, consider hiring a financial planner, taking an online course such as The White Coat Investor's Fire Your Financial Advisor course, or reading some good books on the subject of asset allocation. Links to all of these resources can be found at https://www.whitecoatinvestor.com.

Once you have your investment plan written down, all that is left is to select the investments that go into the plan. One of the easiest, yet sophisticated, investments to use is a mutual fund. A mutual fund consists of a group of investors who pool their money together to hire a fund manager who selects the investments in the fund and manages the money on behalf of the investors. A mutual fund may invest in stocks, bond, or even a type of stock called a Real Estate Investment Trust (REIT). A typical fund may hold dozens or even thousands of different stocks or bonds. The mutual fund structure provides diversification, liquidity, professional management, and the economies of scale available when thousands of investors pool their funds together.

Some mutual fund managers attempt to only select the best stocks or bonds in an attempt to beat the market. Long-term data suggests that this may not be the best idea as these actively managed funds are usually outperformed in the long run, especially after taxes in a taxable account, by passively managed funds called index funds. In these mutual funds, the fund manager simply tries to match the overall market. This is a relatively easy, low-cost task and essentially guarantees the investors will match the market return. Since an index fund is likely to outperform 80–90% of active fund managers in the long run [4], many savvy investors simply avoid actively managed funds all together in favor of index funds.

Using index funds makes implementing your asset allocation very simple. If your investing plan calls for investing 30% of your portfolio into US Stocks, you can simply buy a US Total Stock Market Index Fund with 30% of your money. These funds or something very similar are available in most 401(k)s, in IRAs, and in taxable accounts. You can do the same thing with International Stocks, Small Stocks, Bonds, REITs, and many other asset classes.

Some 401(k)s and most of the major mutual fund companies such as Vanguard, Fidelity, Charles Schwab, and Blackrock make this process even easier. They offer Life Cycle or Target Retirement Funds that are mutual funds composed entirely of a handful of index funds from various asset classes. All the investor needs to do is select their approximate retirement date by buying a fund such as the Target Retirement 2040 Fund. The fund manager takes care of the rest. All the investor has to concentrate on is funding the plan adequately by saving enough money. These funds can be bought in 401(k)s, Roth IRAs, and even taxable accounts as a one-decision investing product. Certainly these are great options for a resident or young attending just getting started investing. While there may be a few better ways to invest, there are thousands of worse ways. This method is broadly diversified, low-cost, and very liquid. It will automatically rebalance and appropriately adjust the amount of risk you take as you approach retirement.

Doctors and other health care professionals who become financially literate will be able to pay off their student loans and eliminate financial worries from their lives. They will be better partners, parents, and physicians. They will enjoy a wonderful career, reduce the risk of burnout and suicide, benefit from a comfortable, dignified retirement, and be able to support their families and favorite charities. The principles of personal finance, business, and investing may not be taught in our medical schools, but that does not mean that doctors cannot and should not learn and apply them in their lives. Doing so will provide the financial freedom that will in turn allow them to approach their professional and personal lives on their own terms.

References

1. Peckham C. Physician debt and net worth report 2016. https://www.medscape.com/features/slideshow/compensation/2016/public/debt-and-net-worth#page=4. Accessed 15 Apr 2021.
2. Kane L. Physician debt and net worth report 2020. https://www.medscape.com/features/slideshow/compensation/2016/public/debt-and-net-worth#page=4. Accessed 15 Apr 2021.
3. Bhutta N. Changes in U.S. family finances from 2016 to 2019: evidence from the survey of consumer finances. https://www.federalreserve.gov/publications/files/scf20.pdf. Accessed 15 Apr 2021.
4. Liu B. SPIVA U.S. scorecard. https://www.federalreserve.gov/publications/files/scf20.pdf. Accessed 15 Apr 2021.

Disability Insurance

10

Tobias Eng

Introduction

In one of Aesop's more popular fables, a magical goose laid one shiny golden egg every morning. The farmer who owned the goose was slowly becoming wealthy, cashing in on the golden eggs each day at the market. Eventually, though, the farmer became impatient. He wanted to get rich faster, so he devised a plan: he would kill the goose, cut her open, and gather all of her eggs at once. Then, he would then sell the bounty of eggs at the market and become rich!

It did not work, of course. When the farmer cut open his prized goose, he found no eggs. Even worse, his precious goose was dead.

This is a fable about greed, but it is also about our most valued asset: our future earning potential. The goose was worth more alive than dead, and not because of anything the goose currently had, but *because of everything that she would have in the future.*

The same goes for you: If you earn $50,000 while you are in final stages of training, and then $300,000 every year for 20 years, you are worth upwards $6 million dollars in future earned dollars.

You are the goose who lays the golden eggs. It is your career and earning potential that will pay for your home, your automobile, and your children's educations. It is your career and earning potential that will pay for your family's vacations and that will fund your retirement accounts.

Chances are, you have insured all of your eggs—you have homeowners insurance, automobile insurance, and if you have valuable artwork or jewelry, you likely have insurance on those as well.

T. Eng (✉)
Northwestern Mutual, Chicago, IL, USA
e-mail: toby.eng@nm.com

© The Author(s), under exclusive license to Springer Nature Switzerland AG 2022

P. K. Louie et al. (eds.), *The Successful Health Care Professional's Guide*,
https://doi.org/10.1007/978-3-030-95950-0_10

Do you have insurance on your income, though? You may have life insurance, and to be certain, you should. But a far greater risk than dying during your wage-earning years is the risk of becoming disabled or incapacitated during your wage-earning years. Truth be told, during the course of your working years, the risk of being injured and needing disability insurance is always higher than the risk of dying and needing life insurance. A female worker who was born in 2000, for instance, has a 19 percent chance of becoming disabled before she reaches the age of 16, but she has only a 4 percent chance of dying before the age of 60. The statistics vary based on age and biological sex, but in every instance, a person is more likely to become disabled before retirement age than they are to die before retirement age [1].

One of the foundational pieces of any risk management plan, then, is long-term disability insurance. Generally speaking, long-term disability insurance pays employees about 60 percent of their salary if they cannot work for an extended period of time due to chronic illness of debilitating injury. It typically kicks into gear when short-term disability insurance expires, which is commonly 90 to 180 days after the short-term coverage began. Some long-term policies provide a few years of coverage, most provide coverage until Social Security Normal Retirement Age (SSNRA).

What are some of the reasons workers need to use their long-term disability policies? Cancer, car accidents, heart attacks, strokes, carpel tunnel syndrome, early dementia: we all know people who have suffered from each of these challenges, which is why long-term disability coverage is considered foundational, particularly for healthcare workers.

The word "foundational" is, in fact, intentional. Likely, if you have ever attended a housewarming party, you have been given a tour whereby the proud new homeowner shows you the enormous walk-in closet in the master suite, the floor-to-ceiling windows, the granite kitchen countertops. Never once, though, has the homeowner said, "You have to check out the foundation!" Yet, a solid foundation is the most important part of the entire home, and any homeowner who has struggled with a weak foundation knows that they would rather have cheap laminate kitchen countertops than a problematic foundation. All of the other above-ground features, bells, and whistles will be torn down if a foundation needs to be replaced.

The same is true of risk management. As a culture, we like to focus on wealth accumulation. We like to show off all of the above-ground features, bells, and whistles of our lives: the shiny cars, the beautiful engagement rings, and the remodeled kitchens. Monthly or at least quarterly, we fix our eyes on our IRAs, 401(k)s or 457 plans. Yet, all of these may crumble to the ground if the foundation is not stable.

Although many healthcare fields are eligible for disability insurance, a large focus is often targeted towards physicians, so this chapter will primarily describe physicians as examples. However, these concepts can be transferred across healthcare fields. The good news for physicians, particularly those in residency, is that unlike other professionals, doctors are afforded special perks with respect to their long-term disability coverage. Yet, many doctors do not seek additional coverage beyond the group long-term disability coverage provided by their employer.

And this can be a missed opportunity to transfer risk and strengthen that foundation. Let's dissect how long-term disability insurance works for physicians, and what you can do to make sure that you take advantage of the best strategies as related to this foundational risk-management coverage.

The Physician Advantage

Most group disability plans will cover only about 60 percent of your income. Residents and fellows can use Beginning and Professional limits to get supplemental long-term disability coverage considering their future income potential rather than their current salary. The amount of supplemental insurance available changes based on specialty.

Another advantage of locking in your supplemental long-term disability policy while you are a fellow or a resident is this: The coverage is portable, meaning that when your transfer hospitals, or move to open your own practice, you can take the policy with you.

The same is not true of employer-sponsored long-term disability, which has consequences beyond simple portability. When you purchase your own supplemental coverage, it is not only portable, but you can also:

- Lock in your age,
- Lock in your current health status, and
- Have the opportunity of adding an Additional Purchase Benefit (APB) option, which if you meet certain requirements, it allows you to increase the benefit at a later date without having to go through another medical screening.

Think of it like this: If you have a group long-term disability benefit through your current employer, the benefit will not carry into your next employer. If that employer does not offer long-term disability, and you want to purchase your own coverage, at that time you will have to go through a medical screening to determine your rate and eligibility.

On the other hand, if you buy your own supplemental coverage while you are in your residency or fellowship, you can take that coverage with you wherever you go. Later, when you have added years to your life, and your health may have changed, you can add coverage (priced at your current attained age) at the medical class rating you initially received. The older you are, the more expensive you are to insure. In general we are more healthy in our youth than we are as we age.

Policy Benefits

Among the most misunderstood aspects of long-term disability coverage are the policy definitions that determine the type of benefits that will payout, and when they will payout. To qualify as totally disabled, a person has to meet the policy's definition of "disabled." Beyond that, sources of income are often at play when considering disability payouts. If a physician is forced to quit working in their field due to a disability, but they can start a career in another field, are they considered disabled? This depends on the policy definition. For instance, let's think about a surgeon who develops a hand tremor. Some group policies will state that if the surgeon is able to earn an income at any job within their education, training, or experience, they are disqualified from receiving coverage. Certainly, a surgeon can still consult with patients (and other doctors) and may be able to secure a job as another medical professional. But their main money-maker—the ability to do surgery—is gone.

Fortunately, individual plans offer great flexibility that allows the definition of "disabled" to be expanded. Though every company provides a slightly different definition of these categories, most policies are broken into one of four categories:

1. A **modified own occupation policy** provides full benefits so long as the physician totally disabled and is not working. Full benefits are discontinued if the physician begins working in an unrelated profession.
2. A **true own occupation policy** would provide full benefits if you are totally disabled (i.e.unable to perform the material and substantial duties of your regular occupation.). (Remember the surgeon with the hand tremor? They would likely receive full benefits under this plan.) The potential benefit of this policy: You will receive full benefits even if you make a higher income in another occupation or specialty. This policy is more expensive than any of the other policies, but for some physicians, it makes sense. If you have, for instance, a patent on a medical device, or if you are an amazing entrepreneur and can run a profitable business regardless of your disability, this policy would allow you to effectively "double dip," receiving both the payout and an unlimited income in a new profession.
3. A **medical own occupation policy** would provide full benefits if you are unable to perform the material and substantial duties of your medical specialty. Once again, the surgeon with the hand tremor would receive full benefits here. However, if they can work in a different occupation, the benefits change.This is generally the best option for doctors who earn money from procedures, such as dentists, surgeons, and other proceduralists.

These definitions are often accompanied with some gray areas, and certain insurance companies have differing definitions, but the following chart is a close representation of what doctors can expect from the four different policies under various scenarios.

	Scenario #1: Partial disability, but doctor is still able to work	Scenario #2: Partial disability, and physician receives a 50 percent reduction In earnings. The physician loses the ability to perform the money-making aspects of his or her job but can still perform other duties.	Scenario #3: Total disability, and not working	Scenario #4: Total disability, and working in an unrelated profession earning the same or less than before the disability	Scenario #5: Total disability, and working in an unrelated profession earning more than before the disability
Modified Own Occupation	Partial benefits	Partial benefits	Full benefits	Benefits payable under a partial claim. Benefit amount offsets based on partial disability earnings made.	No benefit paid
True Own Occupation	Partial benefits	Partial benefits	Full benefits	Full benefits	Full benefits
Medical Own Occupation	Partial benefits	Full benefits – Assuming the insured has met our criteria and discontinued all gainful employment	Full benefits	New disability income earned + disability benefit paid not to exceed the pre-disability income	New disability income earned + disability benefit paid not to exceed the pre-disability income
Most Favorable Policy	All policies are equal under this scenario.	Medical own occupation policy is the most favorable under this scenario.	All policies are equal under this scenario.	True, and medical policies are equally favorable under this scenario. Modified is the least favorable.	True own occupation is the most favorable policy under this scenario.

Riders to Consider

Many policies in the industry will also offer something called a "rider." A rider is an amendment to the terms of the policy, generally with the purpose of adding benefits. Following is a non-exhaustive list of riders to consider adding to an individual life insurance policy. As always, check with your advisors for the options that best fit your needs.

- As discussed earlier, the **Additional Purchase Benefit** rider allows you to increase your medical coverage in the future in tandem with a salary or income increase—without having to go through medical underwriting. This is a great option young professional including residents and fellows. The ideal candidate is one whose income is likely to increase drastically in the coming years. When you have this rider, no matter what happens to your health, you can buy additional coverage when your income increases.
- The **Inflation Protection Rider** increases the monthly payout in accordance with inflation. These riders are generally broken into two categories: (1) The Future Increase Benefit (FIB) allows you to buy more coverage with changes in the CPI; or (2) The Indexed Income Benefit (IIB) allows you to obtain more coverage based on changed in the CPI while you are disable and receiving benefit checks.
- Another rider to consider is the Catastrophic Benefit (CAT) rider. This rider has the same triggers as a Long Term Care policy. This provision provides a second payout in the event that you are totally disabled and CAT disabled. (i.e. suffering from a catastrophic injury that requires long-term care, such as an in-home nurse.)
- When it is necessary, it is well worth the low cost. Though each policy (and each company) is different, this payment generally kicks into gear if the beneficiary has a mental/cognitive impairment (such as early Alzheimer's disease), or if the beneficiary cannot participate in at least the following activities of daily living:
- Bathing
- Dressing and undressing
- Food preparation and feeding
- Functional mobility, such as walking without assistance and moving in and out of a chair
- Use of restroom/maintaining continence
- Transportation

Cost

The cost of long-term disability insurance is determined by several factors: The company providing the insurance, as well as the insured's health, age, gender, and occupation.

Limitations

When searching for long-term disability insurance, be sure to ask your financial advisor about the policy's limitations. Some policies expire after 2 years of payouts, while some extend until the age of 65. Be aware that most policies do not extend long-term disability insurance for longer than 2 years in cases of mental/nervous disabilities, such as drug addiction or depression. This might be particularly concerning to physicians who see motherhood in their futures: though it generally resolves within the first year, post-partum depression can last longer than 2 years. A little less than half of the participants in a 2014 study were still suffering some symptoms of post-partum depression 3 years after birth! [2].

Be aware that Disability insurance policies contain some features and benefits that may not be available in all states. The ability to perform the substantial and material duties of your occupation is only one of the factors that determine eligibility for disability benefits and policies contain exclusions, limitations, and reduction-of-benefits provisions. Eligibility for disability income insurance, additional policy benefits, and qualification for benefits, is always determined on a case-by-case basis.

When Choosing a Policy

When choosing a Disability Insurance Carrier, you are looking for a policy and a company that will be there when you need them. Before settling on a policy, know the answers to these questions:

- What volume of business does the company have in total?
- How much do they pay out in claims?
- What is the company structure? Is it a private, publicly traded or Mutual company?
- Is the policy a modified own occupation, transitional own occupation, true own occupation, or medical own occupation?
  - In other words, how does a company determine what qualifies as a "disability"?
  - How does a company measure "income"? What sources count?
- What is the company's financial strength rating?
- Is the policy non-cancelable? A non-cancelable policy means that premium payments are contractually guaranteed. This is an important guarantee to have if the company has a low financial strength rating.
- Does the policy have a guaranteed renewability provision? This means that the policy must be renewed as long as premiums are paid.

Does the company have a "participating" policy? Some mutual companies will share premium surplus with policy holders via dividends.

Conclusion

We often say that death is the worst possible outcome. It is the worst thing that could happen. It is worst-case scenario. From an emotional point-of-view, death is almost always the worst-case scenario. It is tragic when it happens late in life. An early death? Well, that is almost unspeakable. Your early death is the worst thing that could happen to you, to your family, and to your loved ones. But from a financial perspective, losing your own income during life can be catastrophic, particularly if you are incapacitated. Most physicians have life insurance policies that pay out in the horrific event of an early death, but they often do not have long-term disability insurance. And to be sure, the financial implications can be catastrophic. Medical debt and job loss due to an illness are responsible for more than half of bankruptcies [3].

And what happens if you need ongoing medical care? Not only does your family need to find a way to supplement your income, they also must find a way to pay for your long-term care. Long-term disability coverage helps to insure our income. We wouldn't dream of driving a car with an automobile policy, and the bank won't even allow you to purchase a home without homeowners insurance. You are the goose who lays the golden eggs, so why should your income be any less important?

References

1. Maleh J, Bosley T. Disability and death probability tables for insured workers born in 2000 (p. 3, Rep. No. 20.6). Baltimore: Social Security Administration; 2020.
2. Vliegen N, Casalin S, Luyten P. The course of postpartum depression. Harv Rev Psychiatry. 2014;22(1):1–22. https://doi.org/10.1097/HRP.0000000000000013.
3. American Public Health Association. Medical Bankruptcy: Still Common Despite the Affordable Care Act, Page 432.

Teaching

11

Jona Kerluku, Bryan Aristega Almeida, and Duretti Fufa

History of Medical Education

Hippocrates is credited with being the first physician to use an evidence-based approach to logically assess for a diagnosis and treat patients (Fig. 11.1). Around the 2nd century, Galen built on Hippocratic practices by using animal dissections as a method of understanding human anatomy and improving surgical techniques [1]. Medical advancements and innovations were not restricted by region, and involved further contributions from ancient India, ancient China, and the Middle East [1–7].

Early physicians learned the foundations of medicine through classical texts and depended heavily on master physicians to gain additional skills. However, early medical education was historically unstructured [8, 9]. Physician qualifications to practice medicine independently were solely based on the reputation of the individual. No system yet existed to ensure patients received quality care. Structured methods to create medical practice credentials such as a fixed duration of training or licensing regulations did not develop until the 19th century [10, 11].

Moving forward to medical education in the 20th century, when an educational structure eventually developed in the United States, the Carnegie Foundation funded a quality control analysis called the Flexner Report. This report published in 1910 was a monumental critique on the quality of the medical curriculum and fundamentally shifted the course of medical school curriculums across the nation for upcoming years. The most significant changes included increasing admission and graduation standards [11].

J. Kerluku (✉) · D. Fufa
Hand and Upper Extremity Service, Hospital for Special Surgery, New York, NY, USA
e-mail: kerlukuj@hss.edu; fufad@hss.edu

B. Aristega Almeida
Weill Cornell Medical College, Weill Cornell Medicine, New York, NY, USA
e-mail: baa2019@med.cornell.edu

© The Author(s), under exclusive license to Springer Nature Switzerland AG 2022

P. K. Louie et al. (eds.), *The Successful Health Care Professional's Guide*,
https://doi.org/10.1007/978-3-030-95950-0_11

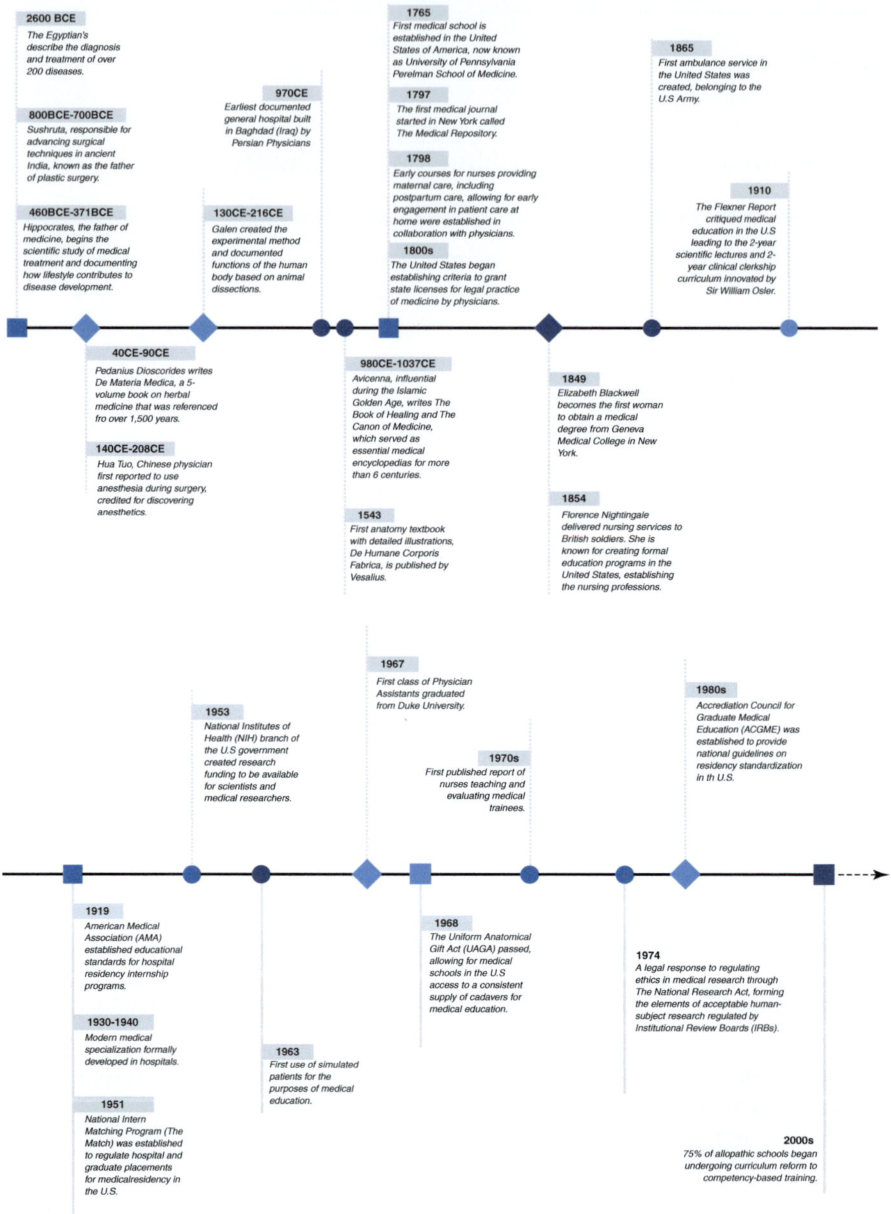

Fig. 11.1 A Short History of Medical Education

Advancements continued shortly after World War I, also contributing to the characteristics of modern medicine still practiced today. The volume of war time causalities caused the nursing profession to restructure, as well as the roles of physician assistants and emergency medical emergency technicians (EMTs) to develop [10, 12, 13]. These professions eventually expanded to civilian medical services in the 1960s. Government support was essential to these expansions and further supported innovations in medicine by developing special funding sources through the National Institutes of Health (NIH).

The restructuring of healthcare delivery and medical education was not only necessary for efficient training but also ensured medical care safety for patients [5]. Recently, medical education is moving toward competency-based training, with increased emphasis on simulated labs. Although medical education is now more structured, learning medicine remains dependent on teaching of medical professionals in the hospital setting through the care of patients. Therefore, the importance of teaching, from early to modern medicine, is inextricably linked to quality patient care.

Principles of Educating the Modern Learner

While drawing from the underpinnings of early and childhood education, adult education inherently addresses a distinct learner. Education of the adult learner must consider not only developmental stage, but also social context. This has become increasingly challenging amidst the growing complexities of society. At the time of this writing, Millennials make up about 35% of the workforce, displacing the "Baby Boomer" generation as the largest living generation [14]. Given this growing population of individuals who will be at the forefront of medicine and healthcare, it is imperative to bridge perceived generational gaps. Educators should seek understanding of differences in expectations, priorities, and learning styles to optimize the educational and mentorship experience of this modern age of learners.

Millennials have been described as confident, optimistic, collaborative, tech savvy, interconnected through social networks, altruistic, and feedback driven [14, 15]. Given the trajectory of technology alongside their development, Millennials are described as more interconnected than previous generations. When it comes to education, they often desire active, engaging, and prefer multimedia forms of learning that extend beyond traditional didactics.

Medical education is challenged by generational differences between modern trainees and their educators. Most of today's medical educators belong to Generation X, (born between 1965 and 1976 and characterized as independent, adaptable, thinkers, self-reliant, skeptical and impatient) and to the "Baby Boomers" generation (individuals born between 1946 and 1964 and characterized by their driven work ethic, competitiveness, self-assurance, resourcefulness and judgmental) [15–17]. The facets of teaching and mentoring presented below have been widely discussed as ways in which educators can optimize their teachings based on the learning preferences of modern learners.

Feedback

Modern learners are feedback driven. However, rather than the once or twice scheduled summative feedback and performance reviews used in many traditional educational spaces, modern learners prefer less structured, regular collegial feedback, so called formative feedback [16, 17]. Modern trainees favor assessments that allow for active, rapid, accessible guidance that caters to fast paced, and engaging forms of learning. They are generally a feedback-seeking, success and improvement driven generation [18].

Goal Setting

Educators should provide modern trainees with clear goals and direction early, but not necessarily in formal ways. Explicit goal setting can focus the learner and bridge the gap expectation and competency [17]. Furthermore, modern learners are not afraid to ask for help unlike prior generations and this open nature makes it important for educators to set explicit goals and expectations. Goal setting, along with relevant and frequent formative feedback that is based on a predefined standard of proficiency or competency, facilitates modern learners' achievement of their goals [14, 17, 19].

Mentorship

The impact of mentorship on career performance is well-documented, leading to more publications, grant funding, career satisfaction and likelihood of serving as mentors themselves [14]. Modern learners welcome help and appreciate personalized mentorship. They reject the fear-based culture of reprimand or shame surrounding failure that is familiar to previous generations. Personalized feedback also allows for closer and direct observation which facilitates the active, hands-on learning process [19]. Modern learners expect mentors to be accessible and flexible, having direct verbal and written communication, emphasizing collaboration, leadership, and professionalism.

Like traditional summative feedback, classic mentoring is often based on infrequent quarterly or semiannually meetings. A more effective mentoring strategy described as "micromentoring" coined by Waljee et al., allows for a coaching-like mentorship experience that is based on defined needs over a shorter time frame. Micromentoring works well with formative feedback and defined goal setting as they serve to provide learners with clear directions to meet those goals [18, 20]. Micromentoring also allow for more real-time in the moment changes to behaviors, attitudes, and actions to better accomplish goals. Though it requires more frequent meetings, micromentoring improves satisfaction and desire for more instantaneous feedback and communication.

Collaboration and Team Based Learning

Modern learners possess vast interconnected networks powered by social media. This contributes to their collaborative nature and desire for team-based learning. Encouraging teamwork and team dynamics has become an essential component of the modern training environment [19, 21, 22]. One method of encouraging collaboration includes peer mentoring to facilitate effective support, academic and mentorship discussions [17]. Furthermore encouraging teamwork helps reduce potential for academic competition, lessens feelings of isolation, and takes advantage of the strengths of individuals to help the whole group as a whole [18]. Compared to previous generations, modern learners are less individualistically inclined. As such, they are best poised to collaborate and welcome team-based learning, which reflects the team-based dynamic utilized in today's practice of medicine. Several additional collaborative learning strategies are described in Table 11.1.

The Role of Technology and Active Learning

The modern generation has grown up amidst an explosive progression of technology. Using technology and the internet, modern learners are able to derive large amount of knowledge in a shorter time period which differs from the customs of previous generations. Social media also allows for rapid continuous peer to peer interactions with large numbers of individuals regardless of physical distance [17]. Platforms such as Twitter can also be used to engage trainees in the learning process. Using instant messaging such as tweets to deliver

Table 11.1 Collaborative Learning Strategies Applied to Modern Medical Education

Collaborative Learning Strategies	Approach
Flipped Classroom	Learners complete pre-recorded lessons prior to lecture. Lecture time is dedicated to activities that promote application of knowledge obtained from individual practice.
Team-Based Learning	Emphasizes pre-class preparation (i.e., reading or test questions) prior to engaging in interactive group discussions. Educator facilitates small groups, encouraging team-based skills.
Just-in-Time Teaching	Lecture time is prioritized for questions and content that addresses gaps in understanding after students complete pre-class preparation. Student responses to pre-tests are reviewed by instructors to guide class time.
Think-Pair-Share	Learners reflect on lecture content or clinical problems in pairs or small groups. Educators then allow students to articulate their interpretations as a method of encouraging individual ideas.
Problem-Based Learning	Learning facilitated through discussion of open-ended, professionally relevant problems in small groups. Educator guides meaningful collaboration to help learners improve clinical reasoning and self-directed learning skills.

teaching points or pearls is one method of providing information to a large number of students that can supplement other forms of learning [15]. Therefore, technology-based, active, and interactive teaching modalities play a role in effective learning. Active learning options include the use of small group sessions, in-person workshops, and simulations. Podcasts, online resources, and websites, virtual or simulated cased-based learning are all options to keep the technology-inclined learner engaged.

One effective model of active learning incorporates the concept of the flipped classroom. This strategy is effective in its use of at-home, web or media based self-directed pre-learning that is then reinforced during in class team discussions, case-based studies and problem solving [15]. With the flipped classroom method, the main role of the teacher is to facilitate discussion, guide through challenging problem solving, and finally to consolidate the main teachings objectives.

While there is no single learning modality or preference that works for all students, an effective teaching framework can still incorporate aspects of various teaching modalities, including more traditional didactics. The healthcare educator should remain open-minded, embracing new teaching styles and modalities of learning and mentoring, while recognizing when traditional practices are appropriate.

Tips for Effective Teaching in Different Settings

Next, we will apply these concepts of modern adult education to the distinct teaching environments for educating healthcare professionals.

Teaching in Lectures

As mentioned, modern learners prefer more active styles of engagement with learning over traditional lectures and didactic sessions. For many educators, accomplishing this represents a major shift from drawing on the files of former presentations and giving a 45–60 min lecture. What we now know is important for meaningful learning to take place is active, effortful and repetitive engagement with the material. Some traditional medical education techniques do employ active and active learning principles including small-group, case-based learning and even the Socratic method. However, several additional teaching strategies can be employed to strengthen lectures and improve both learning and retention. When utilized effectively, the flipped classroom pre-materials may take the form of a traditional mini-lecture and the time during the lecture can be spent engaging actively with the group and with the subject matter, returning only to slides with key concepts.

A template for a lecture that models best practices is outlined here:

Before the Lecture

- *Flipped Classroom*: Pre-materials (recorded and/or reading) sent to learners days in advance of lecture. Content outlines teaching objectives. Materials should be of reasonable length to review (<30 min).
- *Repetition:* Prime learners by beginning lecture with review of key learning concepts.
- *Just-in-Time Teaching*: Learners encouraged to send questions to educator in advance of lecture. Pre-test questions given before or at start of lecture to determine knowledge gaps. At start of lecture, audience response system used to inquire which key learning topics require most review.

During the Lecture

- *Think-Pair-Share*: During lecture, activate learner's recall of pre-materials and experience with clinical topic by asking them to pair and discuss a real-life case they have seen that was relevant to the lecture subject matter. After a couple of minutes paired, ask for 1–2 pairs to share the case they discussed with the larger group. Educator highlights the principles from the case that are relevant to the lecture topic.
- *Active Retrieval*: Interleave standardized, multiple-choice questions through the lecture to reinforce key concepts.
- *Problem-Based Learning*: During lecture, cultivate synthesis and metacognition of subject material by asking learners to generate a multiple-choice exam question. Educator facilitates group discussion key aspects of the question, the correct answer as well as incorrect answers.

After the Lecture

- *Lecture Debrief*: Share the teaching and learning techniques utilized in the lecture with learners in order to teach best practices to the future educators.
- *Spaced Retrieval*: Enhance effortful learning of subject matter by asking learners to recall lecture content some days following the lecture through a quiz, post-test or turning in the multiple-choice exam question described above.

As mentioned, the primary goals are to draw on teaching tools that preview key concepts, allow for spaced recall of those concepts as well as effortful engagement with the material by connecting it to prior experience (case-based learning) and applying information to new situations (quizzing, metacognition). Technology such as creating platforms to store pre-recorded materials and audience response system can be helpful. The move towards digital or virtual lectures also underscores the importance of providing materials in advance. The more familiar with the subject matter learners are, the easier it will be to get them to engage even in virtual settings. Encouraging use of the chat box for asking questions and utilizing break-out rooms to facilitate small group discussions help to increase active learning in the virtual environment.

Teaching in Office and Inpatient Care

Health care providers have been educating learners through patient encounters for centuries. Beyond practicing the professional nuances of interacting with patients, gathering a complete patient history and examination, development of clinical reasoning skills are primary educational goals. For development of both clinical reasoning and procedural skill, it is often assumed that by exposure through repetition, the classic "apprenticeship" model, medical professionals will master the desired skillset. However, through increased understanding of how adults learn and following some guiding principles, healthcare educators can objectively ensure and track progress towards mastery. Some of these guiding principles for educating through patient encounters are summarized below.

- *Expectation Setting* – While there is likely a shared understanding between the educator and learner that demonstrating and improving patient history taking, physical exam, differential diagnosis and treatment plan are desired educational goals, other expectation-setting is often overlooked. The healthcare educator should orient the learner by outlining desired patient flow, introducing the learner to patients and explaining their role. Further, the educator can ask the learner what their prior experience with this patient type is and what they hope to learn. In this way, the educator activates the learner's prior knowledge whether it be through patient encounters, cases, or lectures. By probing the learner to set their own educational goals, it engages them in their learning and gives the educator a preview of what components of the patient encounters to pay particular attention to for later feedback. Further, this kind of inquiry on the part of the educator provides the learner with the sense that the educator will act as a mentor, offering personalized education.
- *Observation* – Where possible, observe the learner interacting with the patient. As will be discussed in the coming sections, feedback is best given based on observed behaviors. Too often in the office and inpatient setting, we base our feedback on learners' oral presentation skills only, missing the critical elements of their professionalism, organization of history taking, skills of physical diagnosis, and ways of responding to patient questions. Several tools for objective evaluation of patient encounters are available and can guide educators in the critical components of these encounters for giving feedback [23].
- *Assessment of Clinical Reasoning Skills* – Development of clinical reasoning requires both analysis and reflection [24]. Oral presentation of the patient encounter gives the educator insight as to the learners' current ability to analyze

and synthesize information. Feedback should be directed at organization as well as content of the presentation with attention to assessment of their analysis of the information. The important step of reflection, commonly summarized in the "Assessment and Plan" component of the oral presentation, can be overlooked. Reflection requires time, particularly for a learner with less experience, and allowing space and time for this reflection is a key component of effective teaching in the office and inpatient settings.

- *Feedback and Evaluation* – Feedback is essential to learning and changing behavior. Feedback is given both informally (during each patient encounter through correcting or re-directing components of the history, physical or differential) as well as formally (outside of the patient encounter). More commonly, the informal feedback can be unrecognized by the learner. Previewing to them that feedback will come in these various forms will increase their awareness that they are receiving feedback even when it doesn't feel like a formal feedback session. If you are involved in formal assessment and evaluation, modern learners will appreciate transparent dialogue about performance. It can feel uncomfortable to provide corrective feedback. However, by utilizing the principles discussed later, giving feedback in a timely fashion, and following feedback by opportunities to repeat performance, it is a powerful tool not only for improving clinical reasoning skills, but also for relationship development between the healthcare educator and learner.
- *Synthesis and Consolidation* – The process of reflection requisite for clinical reasoning should continue beyond the office day or inpatient shift. The educator can foster this consolidation and metacognition by probing the learner to seek connections between the days' and prior experience. Similarly, by inquiring the topics that the learner found most challenging, the healthcare educator can provide guidance for continued reading, can utilize case-based learning to revisit these topics, and should create a plan to re-engage with the learner on these topics in the future. This again provides personalized, learner-driven engagement with their education. It both gives accountability to the learner to continue the learning process, and lets them know the educator is invested in helping them in the process.

Teaching Procedural Skill

In certain medical disciplines, surgical specialties for example, development of procedural skill is as important as development of clinical reasoning. Whereas we have countless tools to evaluate knowledge of clinical diagnoses and appropriate treatment options, we have fewer objective tools to teach and assess procedural skill. Classically, procedural skill was learned through observed practice in the clinical care setting, the *see one, do one, teach one* model. But, in the modern era, an increasing variety of simulation tools are available. The use of simulation has shifted the learning of basic procedural skill from the bedside, or operating room, to the laboratory. As such, the healthcare learner can be expected to obtain or demonstrate appropriate skill there and acquire more complex skills in the more limited patient encounters. In this way, simulation is beneficial not only for patient care and safety, but all for efficiency of education, a concern in the increasingly regulated fields of medical education.

Myriad simulation models and tools for evaluation of competence surrounding procedural skill exist within each medical discipline and are particularly robust in anesthesia, emergency medicine and emergency response, as well as surgical specialties. As important as the fidelity, or characteristics of the simulation tool to approximate real patient setting is the ability to measure learner's performance. Various Observed Structured Assessment Tools (OSATs) exist that can be applied both to the simulated as well as real patient encounters [25]. To review all of these is outside of the scope of this chapter, however guiding principles for effective teaching any type of procedural skill are outlined below.

- *Deliberate Practice* – Learning of all forms, not only of procedural skill, requires repetitive performance. Healthcare learners should be encouraged to practice and given space and time to do so. While practice can be measured in time and repetitions, it can also be made more effective. Learning is more effective when it is effortful. As such, simulation has limitations versus practice in the real-life setting given the stakes and complexity of performance is elevated in real patient care. Aside from the complexity of the procedure, practice can be made more effortful by interleaving practice of different skills as opposed to practicing a singular skill repetitively. Although measured improvement may appear (and feel) easier when the same procedure is rehearsed repetitively in blocks, the long-term gains associated with blocked learning are fewer than when learning is interleaved. This is because the retrieval of skill acquisition is spaced and therefore more effortful. In the practical setting, this means lab trainings should mix various skills acquisition within one session. And perhaps counterintuitively, it also means that learners will get more from practice in an operating room setting where they do one procedure, followed by a different procedure, then return to the original procedure, as opposed to practicing the same procedure three times in a row. The more varied the practice settings, the better as this allows the learner to apply the newly rehearsed skills to varied settings [26, 27].
- *Break skill into smaller steps* – Particularly with more complex procedural skills, to break the skill in to smaller component steps is an effective tool for teaching. While this can be challenging for educators for whom the skill has become to some degree automatic, so called *unconsciously competent,* it is an important tool to communicate and teach effectively (Fig. 11.2). By focusing on a particular step, as opposed to mastery of the complex skill as a whole, both the educator and learner can more easily perceive improvements [28].
- *Apply a framework* – Taking *see one, do one, teach one* to the next level, Walker and Peyton outline the following four step process for learning procedural skills (Table 11.2):

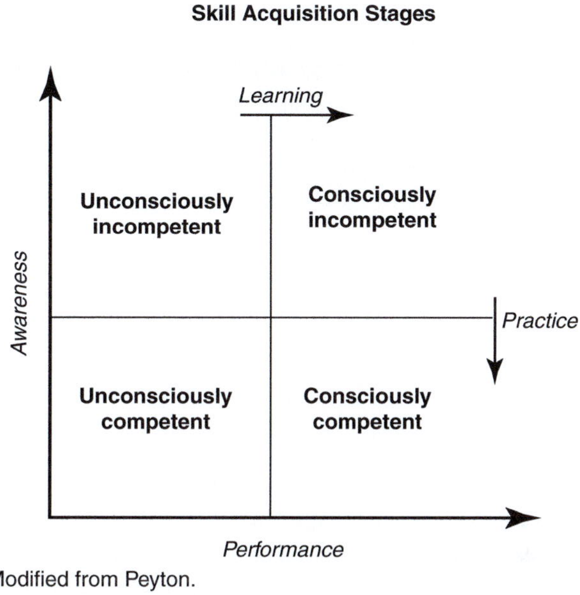

Fig. 11.2 Stages in Skill Acquisition

Table 11.2 Framework for Teaching Procedural Skills

Demonstration	Educator demonstrates at normal speed, without commentary
Deconstruction	Educator demonstrates while describing steps
Comprehension	Educator demonstrates while learner describes steps
Performance	Educator demonstrates while learner describes steps

This framework draws on repetition, breaking the learning process into clear steps as well as uses vocalization to break the procedure down in to steps. It also allows multiple opportunities to confirm comprehension and correct mistakes through the learning process [28].

- *Assessing the learner* – As mentioned, assessment of skill is as important as teaching it. Quality assessment requires direct observation, followed by feedback, paired with opportunities for repeated performance. Assessment paired with feedback assists in the learners' acquisition and retention of skills. As a healthcare educator of procedural skill, recognize that success in this domain includes competence in both knowledge as well as performance. Try to assess where the learner is on the spectrum of *Knowing → Knowing How → Showing How → Doing*. Appreciate that performance (doing) may be improved by reinforcement of earlier stages of the learning process. Assess, *does the learner know the relevant anatomy, the steps? Can the learner vocalize the steps?* If the answer is no, focusing on those learning gaps may be necessary before focusing on practice or performance [29]

- *Importance of objective feedback* – Feedback will be the focus of the final portion of this chapter, but as it relates to teaching procedural skill, tools such as OSATs and review of video-recording of skill performance can be useful adjuncts to traditional oral feedback. These tools add objectivity as well as ability to track improvement over time. Objective and comparative documentation can also assist in identifying learners who are outliers and may need additional practice or support to develop safe and satisfactory procedural skill. Additional strategies for engaging with learners who are struggling will be discussed later.

Creating Space for Teaching with Limited Time

Aside from lack of formal training in how to teach, educators often report pressures of time and clinical productivity as barriers to teaching. While undoubtedly quality teaching in healthcare, as has been described in this chapter, requires not only effort with attention to the needs of the learner, but also requires time. Ideally, quantification of time spent, quality of educator's evaluations, and objective measures of learner development can be utilized to advocate for protected or compensated time for teaching. Unfortunately, in many clinical settings this is not commonplace. Some strategies to facilitate teaching while maintaining forward flow in patient care are summarized below.

- *Scheduling* – on days when working with learners, template patient visits and procedures accordingly. Allowing the learner to spend time with new patients while the educator sees quicker follow-up patients allows ongoing throughput in the outpatient setting. Similarly, planning operative cases to facilitate the stepwise learning of procedural skill outlined above, or putting procedures of appropriate complexity for more junior versus more senior learners together can facilitate the efficiency of learning environment and optimize learners' advancement.
- *Physical examination* – that the educator develops skills of verbalizing aspects of the physical exam while performing maneuvers is critical in helping learners familiarize with abnormal physical findings that cannot be replicated in the simulated setting. This can also facilitate teaching even if the learner is not the one performing the examination. It is helpful to assess patients' comfort level with learners repeating certain portions of the examination. The educator can announce role and training level of the learner and ask patients' permission to incorporate the learner into the encounter.
- *Teach out loud* – instead of providing feedback on the patient encounter outside of the exam room, teach while examining and counseling patient. The educator should be cautious to not suggest that components of the learner examination or counseling had been incorrect, but rather incorporate discussion of the relevant differential diagnosis to standardized counseling of patients about treatment options and alternatives. When done appropriately, this form of teaching out loud during the patient encounter doubles as a powerful tool that enhances communication and facilitates shared decision-making with the patient.

- *Documentation* – turn the dreaded electronic medical record into a tool for teaching. While it is well-established that patients prefer that providers not document during the patient encounter, the learner can be instructed to utilize the time while the educator is counseling the patient to enter key components of the history, physical exam findings and orders. Similarly, summative feedback can be given at the end of a patient care day when the educator is reviewing and signing learners' documentation. While spending the requisite time to countersign these notes, draft an email to the learner that summarizes feedback on patient encounters.
- *Teaching through best practices* – utilize team-trainings and quality initiatives as teaching opportunities. The best practices of pre- and de-briefs at the start and conclusion of a patient day or operative case are perfect opportunities to verbalize expectations, preview critical steps, provide feedback and summarize educational opportunities. The general components of a debrief parallel simple models for feedback including reflecting upon what went well, what could be improved, incorporating multiple perspectives during the process, and synthesizing next steps.

Engaging Diverse Learners

Creating a learning environment where various types of learners can thrive is important. To do this appropriately, educators can familiarize themselves with different learning and communication styles. Two broad personality groups are introverts and extroverts. Introverts tend to prioritize listening over speaking, they prefer to work independently, and enjoy solitude as a way of recharging from social interactions [30, 31]. Extroverts on the other hand, thrive when interacting with others, they prefer to think out loud, and are comfortable with providing on the spot presentations without less time for preparation [32]. There are also those with characteristics on both ends of this the spectrum, known as ambiverts, who do not strongly embody characteristics of either introverts or extroverts [33].

Extroverts tend to be charismatic and outgoing, so they are not often overlooked in group settings. Introverts conversely may struggle vocalizing their thoughts in group conversation, which can lead to their contributions going unnoticed. As a result, introverts can develop a false reputation of being shy, when often all that is needed is a comfortable social setting that allows introverts to contribute to purposeful conversations. Overall, estimates show that 35–50% of people are introverts. By using strategic approaches to encourage participation from all types of learners, educators can substantially improve the learning environment by ensuring all learners' voices are recognized [30, 34].

Specific strategies to facilitate the learning environment for both introverts and extroverts are detailed in Table 11.3. Beyond understanding the personality tendencies of your learners, understanding your own typology and preferred ways of interacting and communicating can also help you become a more effective teacher and mentor to diverse individuals.

Understanding different learning and personality styles not only helps the educator to incorporate better teaching strategies, but it can also help when a learner is

Table 11.3 Approaches to Engaging with Introverts and Extroverts

Learning Environment	Key Learning Style Differences	Approach to Introvert	Approach to Extrovert
Lectures and Didactics	– As adult education moves lectures to more interactive experiences, differences between introverts and extroverts emerge. – Introverts thrive in the classic lecture where they can listen and reflect. – Extroverts on the other hand more commonly thrive in being put on the spot, where they can demonstrate knowledge through external validation.	– Structure lectures and didactics to allow time and space to reflect before posing questions to the larger group (example, *Think-Pair-Share* model). – Create interactive opportunities that allow introverts to draw on their listening skills in facilitating and bringing out diverse reflections on subject matter.	– Incorporate active learning strategies to keep extroverts interested and engaged. – Avoid exceeding 10–15 min of lecture without break for interactive learning.
Small Group Discussions	– Personality differences may result in extroverts dominating small group conversations. – Introverts often require more time to process questions before feeling comfortable to respond. – Seeing extroverts as the first to speak, introverts may not feel there is space to share their thoughts, opinions.	– Preview in advance of the small group session what the discussion questions will be so that introverts can have adequate time to reflect. – Instead of opening questions to the group, call on individuals for their thoughts. – Avoid small groups that are imbalanced in personality type to avoid single dominant personality type.	– If one or two voices begin to dominate group discussion, be sure to guide the group to include more voices. This may include cutting short or redirecting extroverts. – Ask individuals to defend a particular conclusion even if it is not their own opinion – this both diffuses the extroverts' conviction as well as emboldens the introvert who feels less put on the spot to express or defend their own opinion.
Clinical Teaching	– Naturally quicker to participate verbally, extroverts may appear more engaged in the educational process. – Introverts' quiet reflection may be incorrectly perceived as disinterest or having lack of knowledge.	– Be deliberate in drawing out introverts' knowledge with questions. – Make space for opportunities to speak in more private settings.	– Recognize these differences and how you as an educator judge learners' engagement. – Am I creating comfortable space for both types of learners?

(continued)

Table 11.2 (continued)

Learning Environment	Key Learning Style Differences	Approach to Introvert	Approach to Extrovert
Mentorship and Feedback	– Introverts' preference for being behind the scenes can result in less attention from mentors. – Introverts will also have less tendency to self-promote or share accolades. – Extroverts may be easier to engage in feedback dialogue compared to introverts who may prefer more time to reflect in advance of feedback sessions.	– Schedule times to reach out to mentees who are introverts. – Be careful not to perceive introverts' lack of reaching out as lack of need or desire for mentorship. – Highlight and recognize introverts' contributions. – Preview feedback session so that introverts can prepare themselves. – Reserve feedback for private settings, potentially removed from the activity to give increased time for reflection.	– Extroverts will enjoy frequent contact and open dialogue with mentors. – Provide feedback "on the go", proximate to the observed behavior. – Establish mentorship expectations and boundaries to ensure mentor-mentee satisfaction in mentorship relationship.

struggling [35–40]. The pursuit of a career as a healthcare professional is inherently challenging. It is competitive, lengthy, and demanding of both time and emotional energy. When not adequately acknowledged or addressed, these characteristics contribute to emotional exhaustion and burnout in healthcare learners which may substantially impact performance. Objective evaluation and assessment allow educators to detect changes in performance that may be a sign of outside stressors. Such objective evaluation also helps to identify outliers who may benefit from intervention or remediation.

Upon recognition of unsatisfactory performance, initial efforts should try to identify potential causes. Among many possibilities, the learner may be facing personal and professional stressors (i.e. family issues, financial hardships, health concerns, burnout), cognitive differences (such as attention deficit hyperactivity disorder, autism spectrum disorders), or substance abuse problems. Distinct approaches should be employed accordingly. Second, identification of the deficient domain(s) of performance is key. Three core areas of performance include knowledge, skills, and behavior (Table 11.4). Infrequently deficiencies are global across all performance domains and focusing discussion on strengths as well as weaknesses can ease these challenging conversations. Given the multiple challenging aspects of healthcare, it is estimated that 25% of learners may require some form of remediation throughout their training. It is important to normalize hardship, perhaps drawing on personal experience, to make the learner more comfortable in engaging in dialogue [35, 36].

Table 11.4 Strategies to Support Learner Performance in Various Domains

Performance Domain	Examples	Strategies to Support Improvement
Knowledge	Low in-training scores Incomplete or inaccurate patient presentations, diagnoses, plan and documentation Low scores on rotation evaluations	Rule out potential cognitive barriers Inquire about study strategies and offer best practices Establish clear expectations
Skills	Clinical reasoning deficiencies Physical diagnosis, motor, procedural skills deficiencies	Ensure objective assessment is taking place Provide video feedback of performance for self-reflection Provide videos of desired/preferred technique, behavior Ensure knowledge deficits are not driving skills performance gaps, if so, focus first on bridging knowledge gaps Provide opportunities for practice and repeat performance
Behavior	Problems with unprofessional or disruptive behavior Difficulty with timeliness, both at work and with administrative deadlines Strained professional relationships Not receptive to feedback	Recognize that there are multiple perspectives on behaviors and inquire as to the learners' experience Recognize if bias or stereotyping play a role in perception of behavior Censure the behavior, not the individual Offer tools to support organization (technology, coaching) Encourage self-reflection Emphasize accountability for the impact of behaviors on others regardless of the intention Build sense of safety and belonging

After identifying the targeted problem domain(s), another important step to begin these conversations is to assess the learners' insight regarding the perceived problem. After understanding the learner's perspective, the educator or mentor can more effectively meet the learner where they are. It is important to recall that the learner will naturally feel vulnerable and defensive. Starting conversations with inquiry and normalizing feedback, both positive and negative, are powerful tools to build trust that will be necessary to work collaboratively through honest reflection and collaborative development of an action plan.

Learners who are struggling first and foremost need support [36]. Interactions that reinforce feelings of inadequacy or imposter syndrome and emphasize blame or disappointment over inquiry and understanding will have a counterproductive effect on performance. Creating a culture that incorporates regular feedback paired with promoting inclusivity and belonging that is required for psychological safety will increase the likelihood that learners will ask for help when faced with challenges. Supporting learners to persevere through challenges and regain confidence in their performance after such struggles ultimately strengthens the learner-educator/mentor-mentee relationship.

Giving Feedback

Feedback is critical to growth and learning. While educators and learners know this to be true, there are many barriers to quality feedback. This section will both acknowledge the challenges to giving and receiving feedback, while also providing guidance to best feedback practices.

Barriers to Feedback

Ideally, feedback is a two-way conversation that requires reflection from both parties (learner and educator). As previously mentioned, reflection is key to learning, but it requires time. Myriad time constraints are a challenge to meaningful feedback conversations. Because the aim of feedback is to change or improve behavior, conversations surrounding constructive or negative feedback can feel uncomfortable leading to either or both parties avoiding important information exchange. This avoidance may result from fear of undesirable consequences on the relationship. Another barrier to feedback can be absence of clear expectations or standards for competence. As will be discussed, clarifying expectations, like feedback, is a powerful tool to improve performance. A final challenge to giving quality feedback is also insufficient knowledge of tenets of effective feedback. These will be reviewed in the remainder of this section.

Effective Feedback

Feedback can be given in multiple forms, but grossly can be categorized as *formative* or *summative*. Formative feedback is akin to coaching, given in real time and proximate to the observed behavior. Summative feedback is more commonly given at the end of an educational block or experience, these may be in the form of end-of-rotation debriefs or evaluations. Both forms of feedback are important. All too often, formative feedback, which is less formal, can be overlooked. Every educational experience provides an opportunity to give and solicit feedback. Self-reflection should be encouraged. When the educational experience will last some time, such as a clinical rotation, it is best practice to meet with a learner at the beginning of a rotation to establish educational objectives, solicit the learner's prior experience, goals and areas for desired growth as well as to establish clear expectations including how feedback will be given. To repeat this process at the mid-way point allows both parties to communicate on progress while there is still time to modify approaches. Finally, end-of-rotation feedback reviews previously established goals, progress, and plans for future.

Beyond building an expectation and cadence for giving feedback, it can remain difficult to know how and on what it is appropriate to give feedback. Stated briefly, feedback should report on observed and modifiable behaviors. This means avoiding giving feedback on personality characteristics, such as being "shy", "confident". Feedback should give the recipient the opportunity to reflect on their performance,

Table 11.5 Basics of Giving Feedback

When?	Timely relative to the observed behavior Observed behaviors are fresh in mind of both feedback giver and receiver
Where?	Safe, quiet, private environment Ideally disengaged from the task to give feedback Most commonly not in front of patients or colleagues, particularly if corrective
How?	Reports on specific, firsthand, objective information Use descriptive, not evaluative language Regulated in quantity and limited to modifiable behaviors Accompanied by explanations Reinforces positive performance and behaviors Provides guidelines for improvement Includes an action plan and opportunity for follow-up

while the feedback giver both reinforces desired behaviors and provides guidelines for improvement. Finally, feedback should provide a plan and opportunity for repeated performance (Table 11.5).

Multiple templates and frameworks for giving feedback exist. Common themes between frameworks include previewing to the receiver that you are about to offer feedback, gaining insight as to the receiver's perception of the performance by asking how they think it went (both positive and negative), reporting objectively on a specific behavior including explaining the desired alternative behavior where relevant, and concluding by offering encouragement and support in ongoing growth.

Feedback and the Growth Mindset

Author and researcher Carol Dweck describes the growth mindset as the assumption that abilities can be developed, as opposed to ability being innate. Mastery occurs through dedication and hard work, which fosters a love of learning and resilience that is essential for highest levels of accomplishment [41]. Feedback can be a tool to foster a growth mindset in our learning environments. By focusing on improvements over simply results, growth-oriented feedback praises the learning process and effort to improve performance. Some simple strategies to giving growth-oriented feedback include:

- Praising the process
- Recognizing effort as a positive attribute, not as a sign of lack of ability
- Focusing on effort over complimenting innate intelligence
- Focusing on improvements rather than results
- Inserting the word "yet" – *"Your physical exam skills are not **yet** where I expect them to be at this stage of the rotation"*

Feedback provides an important opportunity to reinforce positive behaviors as well as to learn from and grow beyond behaviors that do not align with clinical competence. It is a vital component of being an effective teacher and healthcare educator. Learners can be coached to receive feedback with a growth mindset as well, reinforcing that skills and knowledge improve through effortful learning, focusing on getting better rather than being good, and viewing feedback as an opportunity for personal and professional development. In this way, receiving feedback shifts fear of judgement to meaningful growth. As the American poet, Archibald McLeish said, "The only one thing more painful than learning from experience is not learning from experience".

Summary

Parallel with other medical advances, modern medical education has advanced tremendously as we have improved understanding of how adults learn. Effective healthcare educators should seek to make teaching active and personalized. Traditional hierarchies within medicine should move towards collaborative conversations. More than ever, diverse individuals are pursuing careers in healthcare. Effective communication across a variety of learners will increasingly incorporate technology and frequent feedback. Cultivating a culture rooted in the growth mindset praises effort over performance and helps build resilience important to the lifelong learning required of healthcare professionals.

References

1. Hajar R. History of medicine timeline. Hear Views. 2015;16(1):43.
2. Hua Tuo | Chinese physician and surgeon | Britannica. Available from: https://www.britannica.com/biography/Hua-Tuo
3. The islamic roots of the modern hospital – AramcoWorld. Available from: https://www.aramcoworld.com/Articles/March-2017/The-Islamic-Roots-of-the-Modern-Hospital
4. Ghosh SK. Human cadaveric dissection: a historical account from ancient Greece to the modern era. Anat Cell Biol. 2015;48(3):153–69.
5. Holt DA, Sinnott JT, Van Sant SP, Behnke RH, Lipp K. A medical history timeline. J Fla Med Assoc. 1993;80(2):121–3.
6. Champaneria MC, Workman AD, Gupta SC. Sushruta: father of plastic surgery. Ann Plast Surg. 2014;73(1):2–7.
7. Gurunluoglu R, Gurunluoglu A. Paul of Aegina: landmark in surgical progress. World J Surg. 2003;27(1):18–25.
8. Dezee KJ, Artino AR, Elnicki DM, Hemmer PA, Durning SJ. Medical education in the United States of America. Med Teach. 2012;34(7):521–5.
9. Custers EJFM, Ten CO. The history of medical education in Europe and the United States, with respect to time and proficiency. Acad Med. 2018;93(3):S49–54.
10. Riesenberg LA, Little BW, Wright V. Nonphysician medical educators: a literature review and job description resource. Acad Med. 2009;84(8):1078–88.
11. Fee E. The first American medical school: the formative years. Lancet. 2015;385(9981):1940–1.
12. JI MK. Historical review of emergency medical services, EMT roles, and EMT utilization in emergency departments. J Emerg Nurs. 1985;96(3):414–23.
13. Americannursing:anintroductiontothepastnursing,history,andhealthcarepennnursing.Available from: https://www.nursing.upenn.edu/nhhc/american-nursing-an-introduction-to-the-past/
14. Louie M, Moulder JK, Wright K, Siedhoff M. Mentoring millennials in surgical education. Curr Opin Obstet Gynecol. 2019;31(4):279–84.

15. Hopkins L, Hampton BS, Abbott JF, Buery-Joyner SD, Craig LTB, Dalrymple JL, et al. To the point: medical education, technology, and the millennial learner. Am J Obstet Gynecol. 2018;218(2):188–92. https://doi.org/10.1016/j.ajog.2017.06.001.
16. Barmparas G, Imai TA, Gewertz BL. The millennials are here and they expect more from their surgical educators! Ann Surg. 2019;270(6):962–3.
17. Chen PH, Scanlon MH. Teaching radiology trainees from the perspective of a millennial. Acad Radiol. 2018;25(6):794–800. https://doi.org/10.1016/j.acra.2018.02.008.
18. Meister JC, Willyerd K. Mentoring millennials. Harv Bus Rev. 2010;88(5):68–72.
19. Desy JR, Reed DA, Wolanskyj AP. Milestones and millennials: a perfect pairing—competency-based medical education and the learning preferences of generation Y. Mayo Clin Proc. 2017;92(2):243–50. https://doi.org/10.1016/j.mayocp.2016.10.026.
20. Waljee JF, Chopra V, Saint S. Mentoring millennials. JAMA. 2020;323(17):1716–7.
21. Barnds WK. Millennials invading: building training for today's admissions counselors. Coll Univ. 2009;85(2):63–6.
22. Roberts DH, Newman LR, Schwartzstein RM. Twelve tips for facilitating millennials' learning. Med Teach. 2012;34(4):274–8.
23. Pelgrim EA, Kramer AW, Mokkink HG, Van den Elsen L, Grol RP, Van der Vleuten CP, et al. In-training assessment using direct observation of single-patient encounters: a literature review. Adv Health Sci Educ Theory Pract. 2011;16:131–42.
24. Koharchik L, Caputi L, Robb M, Culleiton AL. Fostering clinical reasoning in nursing students. Am J Nurs. 2015;115(1):58–61. Available from: https://journals.lww.com/ajnonline/Fulltext/2015/01000/Fostering_Clinical_Reasoning_in_Nursing_Students.31.aspx
25. Mansoorian MR, Hosseiny MS, Khosravan S, Alami A, Alaviani M. Comparing the effects of objective structured assessment of technical skills (OSATS) and traditional method on learning of students. Nurs Midwifery Stud. 2015;4(2):27714. Available from: /pmc/articles/PMC4557410/
26. Harris KR, Eccles DW, Shatzer JH. Team deliberate practice in medicine and related domains: a consideration of the issues. In: Advances in health sciences education, vol. 22. Cham: Springer; 2017. p. 209–20. https://doi.org/10.1007/s10459-016-9696-3.
27. Brown PC. Make it stick. Cambridge/London: Harvard University Press; 2014. https://doi.org/10.4159/9780674419377.
28. Peyton R, Harris MWD, Morrison R, Allery RPL, Harris D, Peyton LPR, et al. Teaching and learning in medical practice 1998.
29. Burgess A, van Diggele C, Roberts C, Mellis C. Tips for teaching procedural skills. BMC Med Educ. 2020;20(2):1–6.
30. Lebin LG, Riddle M, Chang S, Soeprono T. Continuing the quiet revolution: developing introverted leaders in academic psychiatry. Acad Psychiatry. 2019;43(5):516–20.
31. de Jongh R, de la Croix A. 12 tips to hear the voices of introverts in medical education … and to improve the learning climate for everyone. MedEdPublish. 2021;10:107.
32. Cullen-Lester KL, Leroy H, Gerbasi A, Nishii L. Energy's role in the extraversion (dis)advantage: how energy ties and task conflict help clarify the relationship between extraversion and proactive performance. J Organ Behav. 2016;37(7):1003–22.
33. Davidson IJ. The ambivert: a failed attempt at a normal personality. J Hist Behav Sci. 2017;53(4):313–31.
34. Colley SL. Equitable education for introverts: providing learning opportunities that prepare nursing students to be leaders. Nurse Educ. 2018;43(5):224–6.
35. Melia MT, Paez A, Reid G, Chirch LM, Luther VP, Blackburn BG, et al. The struggling infectious diseases fellow: remediation challenges and opportunities. Open Forum Infect Dis. 2020;7(3):ofaa058.
36. Merriam SB, McNeil MA, Spagnoletti CL. A 5-step framework for the assessment and remediation of a struggling medical learner in the clinical environment. South Med J. 2019;112(3):135–6.
37. Ridinger H, Cvengros J, Gunn J, Tanaka P, Rencic J, Tekian A, et al. Struggling medical learners: a competency-based approach to improving performance. MedEdPORTAL. 2018;14:10739.

38. Margolis RD, Ku CM. The "Difficult Learner" in anesthesiology: challenges, pitfalls, and recommendations. Paediatr Anaesth. 2021;31(1):92–102.
39. Crannell WC, Brasel KJ. Dealing with the struggling learner. Surgery. 2020;167(3):523–7.
40. O'Neill LD, Norberg K, Thomsen M, Jensen RD, Brøndt SG, Charles P, et al. Residents in difficulty-just slower learners? A case-control study. BMC Med Educ. 2015;14(1):1–9.
41. Dweck C. Mindset: the new psychology of success. Random House Digital, Inc; 2015.

Leadership Lessons from History

12

Todd J. Albert

Introduction

Leadership is an incredibly popular topic in business schools, management classes and airport bookstores. A google search of the word "leadership" yields 2,520,000,000 citations. In this chapter we will explore elements and important principals of leadership though the lens of history and some of the most notable leaders throughout history. As trainees in the healthcare realm, what lessons can be learned from historical figures spanning across multiple generations and walks of life?

Definition

To discuss leadership, it is best first to define it. While there are multiple definitions of leadership throughout history, an excellent definition is that described by the American Orthopaedic Association: "The art and science of developing, promoting and implementing a practical vision and goals through unselfish and responsible motivation and skill for effective group action." This definition is excellent because it encompasses so many parts of what makes leaders who they are and describes many of the great leaders throughout our history. Unselfishness involves caring more about the group than about oneself. Motivation for group action is critically important and entails great communication skills, promotion of a vision, and assembling the right team and placing each team member in the correct position to effect that successful group action. Basically, the concepts within the definition are creating the vision, setting forth the goals, and aligning the group.

T. J. Albert (✉)
Department of Orthopaedic Surgery, Hospital for Special Surgery, Weill Cornell Medical College, New York, NY, USA
e-mail: albertT@hss.edu

© The Author(s), under exclusive license to Springer Nature Switzerland AG 2022

P. K. Louie et al. (eds.), *The Successful Health Care Professional's Guide*,
https://doi.org/10.1007/978-3-030-95950-0_12

Many people have questioned whether leadership is important and most people who have led (and are students of history) understand that no one person is an island and that no matter how small the group, effective leadership makes whatever the goal within the group is, more attainable and successful. Anyone reading this, especially if they are in or entering the health professional field understands that there are multiple groups within that field whether it be a laboratory group working together, a study group, a group of trainees and/or residents on a floor, a division in a medical specialty, a department in a medical specialty within a school or a hospital, or a group of administrators. Within a business there are also different groups that function to make a business successful. As such, within these groups, whether small or large, leadership is essential.

We live in a world full of disruption. Whether it be in the medical world with consolidation of healthcare markets, changes in the way insurance companies work, disparity between uninsured and under-insured people, or in the broader world having just lived through a pandemic or the social unrest and economic disparities. Now, more than ever, is a time to both understand and search out leaders at multiple levels. As such, this is a reminder that in all aspects of life, leadership is required. As Larry Mathis, a well- known medical leader said, "There is nothing in a healthcare professional's education and training, that qualifies them to be a leader…they are consummate professionals , the best and the brightest. But, when they leave the confines of medicine, they can be a danger to themselves and others." This is perhaps less true now than when the quote was said, but it does point out that there is a yearning need for additional leadership training at an early time in the healthcare career. And even moreso, leadershio should be a critical component of the education during these formative years.

Leaders set an example with behavior, take responsibility, communicate well and listen well, and care more about others' success than their own. Leaders are both teachers and mentors. They are positive, passionate, focused on a mission, and always strive to do the right thing.

In Jim Colllins' book *GOOD TO GREAT*, he performed a data-driven analysis of "transitional" companies. He looked at 11 companies (Abbott, Circuit City, Fannie Mae, Gillette, Kimberly Clark, Kroger, New Core, Philip Morris, Pitney Bowes, Walgreens and Wells Fargo) and did a case control study to determine why they were different. He found that all 11 successful companies had "Level 5″ leaders. These level 5's can be defined as "an individual who blends extreme personal humility with intense professional will." There is a pyramid of leadership whereby Level 1 leaders are highly capable individuals and Level 5 leaders are that type of leader who demands superb results, has unwavering resolve, has vision of true greatness and takes responsibility for failure (Fig. 12.1). Level 5 leaders have personal humility: they are modest, they avoid adulation, they have inspired standards and not necessarily inspiring charisma. They focus on the organization and not on themselves, and they set their successors up for success. Level 5 leaders can be viewed as a window and a mirror. When Level 5 leaders are successful they look outward and sideways through the window to see what they can do further or who they can congratulate and give credit to. Any failure

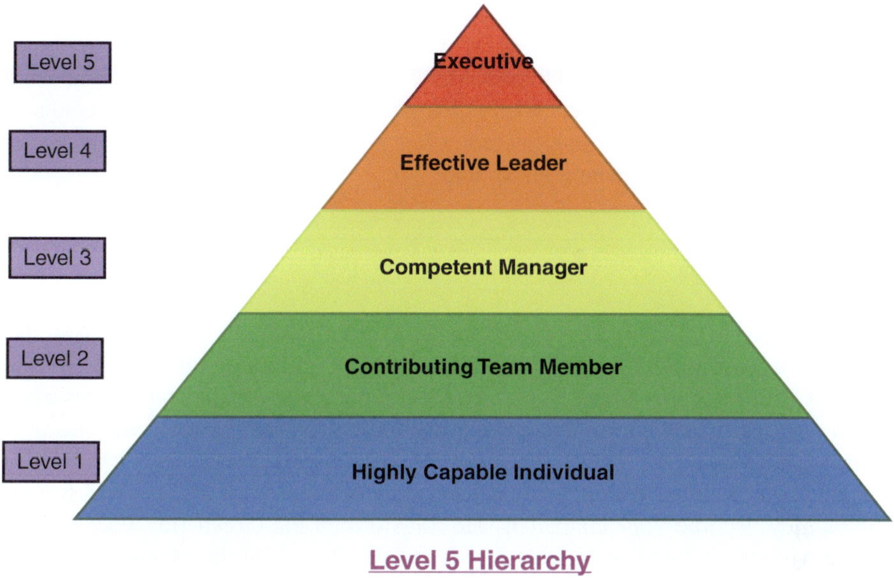

Fig. 12.1 The Leadership Pyramid

becomes the mirror whereby they only look at themselves and what they could have done better.

Two-thirds of the comparison companies in Collins' study had CEOs who were Level 4 leaders. That is, they had gargantuan personal egos, they set themselves up for success and not the company. They typically set up their successors for failure. Those companies did not have long-term success.

An ongoing question is whether anybody can become a Level 5 leader? No one specifically knows this answer. There is no ten step program, but the best advice is to imitate and study those special Level 5 leaders. Another important trait of Level 5 leaders is that they put the right people on the bus. In other words, they hire the correct people and assign them important roles to make the group function better. If those in certain seats on the bus are not functioning, they either are moved to a better seat within the company or moved out if they don't fit with the needs and appropriate talents of the company. Good leaders face the facts. They seek out the truth even if it is not pleasant. They create a culture where honest and open debate thrives. Leaders with strong personalities can unintentionally discourage open communication, which is critical. Accepting the facts allows for appropriate analysis and action. When mistakes are made, postmortems can occur without blame. There is a well-known story to this point of a lower level engineer at Intel, who made a mistake that cost the company over 10 million dollars. The engineer went to speak to the CEO of Intel at the time and said that he was sure that the CEO was going to fire him. The CEO said, "Why would I fire you? I just spent 10 million dollars on your education." This gets to the point of looking for teachable moments. Great leaders look for and exploit teachable moments.

As stated above, one can learn so much and become a better leader by studying those who have a tremendous leadership history. There are great examples in history and hence, the purpose of this chapter. Many examples of great leaders come from sports, the military and politics. While there are countless examples and personalities we could have shared and explored, a few great examples follow to make specific points relative to excellent leadership.

Vince Lombardi

Vince Lombardi was perhaps the greatest American football coach in history. He coached 10 seasons with a career record of 105 wins, 35 losses and six ties. He won five NFC titles and two Super Bowls. There are many great leadership quotes associated with Vince Lombardi. "Winning is a habit. Watch your thoughts, they become your beliefs, watch your beliefs, they become your words. Watch your words, they become your actions. Watch your actions, they become your habits. Watch your habits, they become your character." He transformed the Green Bay Packers into instant winners and was acclaimed the Man of the Decade in the 1960s.

He led the Packers to 89 wins, 29 losses and 4 ties, five NFC titles, and the first two Super Bowl crowns in 9 years. He also led the 1969 Redskins to the first winning record in 14 years. He never had a losing season and was known as a tough task master. Notable about Lombardi is that he started at the age of 45. At that age, many great football legends had already made their mark and many felt it was a younger man's game. He famously said, "Gentlemen, we are going to relentlessly chase perfection knowing full well we will not catch it, because nothing is perfect. But, we are going to relentlessly chase it because in the process, we will catch excellence." This exemplifies a determined leader that wants to inspire those he leads into being the best that each person can be. It demonstrates an important quality of great leaders, maximizing potential in all.

Alexander the Great

Another example of leadership is in the category of great military and/or political leaders. Alexander the Great was perhaps one of the best known historical characters of military leadership. Although he reigned as the King of Macedonia for less than 13 years, Alexander the Great changed the course of history. Known as one of the world's greatest military generals, he created a vast empire that stretched from Macedonia to Egypt and from Greece to part of India. This conquest allowed the Hellenistic culture to become widespread. He was a visionary and enjoyed tremendous loyalty of his troops. He was the son of Philip II and Olympias (one of Philip's seven or eight wives). He was brought up with the belief that he was of divine birth. His mother, from birth, encouraged him to believe that he was a descendent of heroes and gods. He had great charisma and a force of a personality, but his character was full of contradictions especially in his later years (his early '30's). He had abilities to motivate his army to do what seemed to be impossible (according to Susan Abernathy, the freelance history writer in Live Science). Most importantly, Alexander's example of dreaming, planning and strategizing on a large scale as well as motivating his men to win battles even when outnumbered in some of the greatest conquests in history; exemplify that of a leader who leads from the front. He was known to be inspiring and courageous, devoted to training his men and rewarding them with honors and spoils, and going to battle beside them which furthered their devotion and confidence.

Alexander learned much from his father, who campaigned aggressively, but was away quite a bit. His father had Alexander tutored by Aristotle in logic, philosophy, music and culture. Those teachings of Aristotle apparently helped him as he formed his treatment of his new subjects and the empires he invaded and conquered allowing him to admire and maintain these disparate cultures. Alexander's success as a leader is partly a bi-product of his father giving him significant responsibility at quite a young age. The father left Alexander at age 16 in charge of Macedonia while he was away on campaign. Alexander at that time took the opportunity to defeat the Thracian people called the Maedi and founding "Alexandroupolis" a city named after himself. Alexander's father, Philip II, was assassinated in 336 BC, while celebrating his daughter's wedding. At the time of his death he was planning to invade Persia. This aspiration was passed on to Alexander by his mother, Olympias. After his father's death, Alexander quickly consolidated his power and gained support of the Macedonian army. He ultimately invaded Persia and conquered it. Alexander died in 323 BC, after catching a fever while in Babylon. A common mistake made by leaders, and one made by Alexander, is lack of a succession plan. The void left after his death led to some fighting among his generals, but ultimately the conquered territories were divided up. His most significant legacy was the extent and proliferation of great culture that was largely due to Alexander. His greatest leadership traits were his bravery, charisma, fighting beside and in front of his men and his motivational talents.

George Washington

Another great military exemplar is George Washington. People often ask why was George Washington a great leader? Probably five facts inherent to George Washington are true and informative of what can help all of us, as we strive to be better leaders:

1. He was a man of faith and action. He believed deeply in God's providence and demonstrated it in his actions. He was not a man who made eloquent speeches or retreated to the comforts of a tent while the troops were out battling. He, like Alexander, fought alongside his troops and had a history of being a soldier's soldier. He exemplified the saying that "A leader walks the talk." He believed that every leader was the steward of power that was the authority deemed by God and had to act in accordance with that.

2. He demonstrated great character and conviction. Integrity is an important characteristic of any leader and it was exemplified by Washington. By no means was he perfect. He did try to live by words and principles at all times. He had high moral character and this helped him lead the troops during difficult times. The most difficult perhaps being the winter at Valley Forge in 1777 and 1778, when they were outnumbered and losing many battles.
3. He treated those he led with great dignity and respect. He very much valued individual freedoms, he never acted as a tyrant and he extended that freedom to others. He had great faith in those he led and exemplified that which we noted earlier caring much more about those he led than about himself. He treated his troops with great respect.
4. He held high expectations for both himself and those he led. The troops, knowing that Washington had respect for them and that he was vested in their mission, responded by being quite dedicated to him and willing to do all they could for the general. This relationship is quite instructive in demonstrating to leaders how to gain loyalty from those who are following them. A less successful leadership tactic is to set up rules without strong relationships. Also living by the rules as an example is quite helpful.
5. Finally, Washington placed the people's welfare above his own and nothing can create a stronger loyalty than this. When the troops know that a leader truly cares about them, it creates a significant loyalty and dedication that is demonstrative of great servant leadership. The great picture of Washington in the front of the boat crossing the Delaware exemplifies many of these traits that are instructive on leadership (Fig. 12.2).

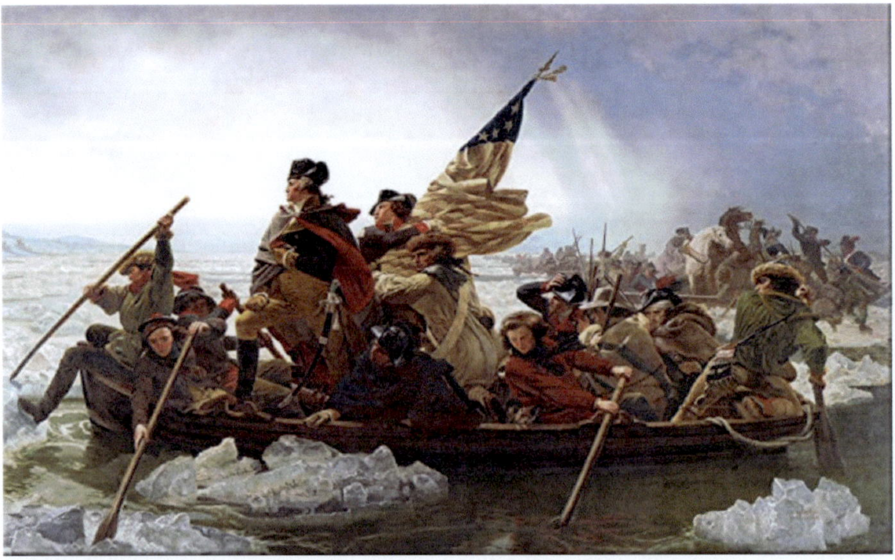

Fig. 12.2 Washington crossing the Delaware

Winston Churchill

Another example of tremendous leadership both in government and in the military is Winston Churchill. He was voted the greatest Britain of all time out of a hundred candidates by the BBC in 2002, and the case for him being the best was powerful. He was first a government minister in 1908 and occupied most of the top jobs in politics during the first half of the century. He retired ultimately in 1955, having served as Prime Minster for 9 years. What really catapulted Churchill to top position as a leader, and in his credit, is his extraordinary leadership in World War II. He was described as bold, brave and tireless in his resolve to take on the might of Nazi Germany. While all others around the world thought Britain's loss was inevitable, Churchill persevered. He was felt to be most powerful in his leadership through rhetoric, but it is well known that his extensive knowledge and pursuit of facts in all decisions was quite helpful during that time. Despite the amazing leadership and his responsibilities and victory in World War II importantly gaining American alliance in the fight against Hitler, he was also known to have made huge mistakes in his long political life. These include Gallipoli and in putting Britain on the gold standard while he was Secretary of the Exchequer in the 1920s. Many thought that convering to the gold standard was a major factor in bringing about the Great Depression. In the 1930s he was an aggressive opponent of Indian nationalism and he also supported Edward VIII during the abdication crisis of 1936.

The six best leadership traits that we can learn from Sir Winston Churchill and that are exemplified in many great leaders, but perhaps demonstrated in Churchill's leadership both during crisis and throughout his life were:

1. Communication
2. Reputation
3. Passion
4. Vision
5. Courage
6. Action

Each of these traits could be the subject of an entire book, but are worth contemplating and studying with regard to Winston Churchill as well as other great historical figures and their demonstrated leadership. All are important and intertwined. Consider these traits as we consider leadership and improvement in the tactics used to formulate how one chooses to lead.

The Stoics

Another group of incredible historical leaders teaching lessons comes from stoicism and the stoics. These historical figures living before and around the birth of Christ, can teach us so much about learning and living in times of leadership, but mostly in times of difficulty, challenges, and crisis. The leadership of many stoics is informative and their communication is incredibly important. Seneca, while not always thought of as a leader, had to learn tremendous leadership in his role as a counsel. Epicteus started as a slave, but became a leader in the stoic school. Zeno, one of the original great stoics, ran a huge shipping empire and had to obviously have tremendous communication and leadership skills in doing that. Cato was a senator, as well as leading troops in battle.

There are many lessons that these and other stoics have taught regarding great leadership. For example, one of the lessons of the stoics is to focus on that which one can control and where one can have influence. Whether a leader, a middle manager, or the leader of only a small group, one should focus on that which they can have an influence on and realize that they can provide opinions and thoughts to people, but that can only go so far in terms of their acceptance of the advice and counsel. Anyone can lead the horse to water, but only a few can encourage them to drink.

Yet another leadership lesson is to never act rashly. There is a difference between rashness and boldness. John F. Kennedy, Jr. said that time is a tool, not a couch. This was put into practice during the Cuban missile crisis to lead with boldness versus recklessness. The great stoic Zeno said, it is better to trip with your feet than your tongue. An important concept in leadership is to never feel that we have to act so quickly. Acting too quickly can lead to mistakes (actions or verbal) that is irretrievable. Looking for teachable moments is also an important aspect of leadership. When people make mistakes, others should accept them and use them to teach and insure that they become better team members and better contributors to overall goals and vision.

Bringing this back to the realm of training to become a healthcare professional, how does one put together so many lessons from history, from leaders in history and from the stoics? There were likely ten stoic philosophies that come from the greatest stoic leader, Marcus Aurelius, who led an empire and remained humble, thoughtful and created one of the best books about stoicism that was not necessarily meant for public consumption, but was written as his own diary of thought: **Meditations**. The ten concepts that come from this school of thought that can be helpful in life and leadership are:

1. Memento Mori – remember you will die. The thought is to live every day as if it's your last both in terms of cherishing the day, but also enjoying the day.
2. Concentrate like a Roman. Tasks that we are both assigned and take on we should perform as if they are the last thing we are ever doing and put our highest concentration effort into those tasks.
3. Amor Fati – love everything. The concept behind this saying is that when good things happen love them. When bad things happen, love them. We can't always control them, but learn from the bad things and learn from the good things.
4. Tame your temper. It has been said that not taming your temper or acting too fast in the face of anger is like returning a bite to a dog. We don't want to regret our actions afterwards so we should hold our tongue. That said, sometimes we

can use temper as a tool. It is possible to feign anger as sometimes we see sports coaches do. Generally, we should control our temper to the best of our abilities.
5. Build a routine. We are what we repeatedly do. This is akin to spending 10,000 hours to become an expert in something, but we should routinely do things to make our lives efficient and excellent in leadership.
6. Always stay a student. We should be humble and inquisitive and understand that we can't learn what we think we already know, so if we remain humble in what our knowledge base is and seek always to learn more we will be more knowledgeable on the other end.
7. Get up early. Marcus Aurelius said do what you were born to do. There is a well- known portion of his book, Meditations, where he is having an argument with himself, convincing himself to awaken and make the most of the day.
8. Accept this moment. As was famously said, at this moment use: (a) objective judgment; (b) unselfish action; and c) willing acceptance. A stoic person does all three of these and accepts that we can't necessarily control outside events, only our response to them.
9. Guard your character. If you live your life with wisdom, temperance, judgment and courage you will protect your character, live a good life and as Marcus Aurelius would say, our actions only ruin our life if they ruin our character.
10. Seize the day. Epicteus was reported to have said that fools have only one thing in common, they all put off living. In other words, tied to the theory of Memento Mori, do not wait for something to happen or act in a way as if life today isn't the best life we can have. Make life the best it can be and accept what comes from that.

Conclusion

There is much to be learned from being inquisitive, studying great leaders throughout history as one defines their own goals for leadership and actions in life. Do understand that there are certain inherent and learned traits which make great leaders great. However, as trainees, there are ample opportunities to practice the art and science of good leadership and behave appropriately as great leaders do, which will ultimately help whatever organization or group following graduation.

Selected Reading

Alexander the Great: Facts, Biography & Accomplishments by Owen Jarus – Live Science.
Aurelius M. Emperor of Rome, long G. *meditations*. Mineola, NY: Dover; 1997.
Collins JC. Good to great. New York: Harper Collins; 2001.
Holiday R. The obstacle is the way. New York: Penguin Group; 2014.
Mathis LL. The Mathis maxims: lessons in leadership. Houston: Leadership Press; 2001.

Generalization vs. Specialization

13

Rick W. Wright

The question of generalization versus specialization in medicine reflects a question that has been raised in earnest over the last decade across a variety of activities and professions in society. The intuitive mindset regarding this topic is impacted by the biases brought to the topic by an individual and may not reflect many of the nuanced issues regarding this topic. In this chapter, I hope to approach this from a variety of angles to allow the reader to more deeply understand and explore what is a relatively complex question/issue.

As explained in an analogy regarding career generalization versus specialization, Anna Matteo used the example of a sushi restaurant [1]. You would expect that a restaurant that specializes in sushi, and prepares no other types of food, to demand and expect higher prices than a restaurant that serves pizza, tacos and sushi. Likewise, you would expect the quality of sushi at a specialized restaurant to be higher. The counter argument as noted in her article is that it must be taken in the context of location and opportunities. Potentially, in a small town, a sushi expert may provide outstanding quality, but the demand is such that they must also offer many other food types to have adequate business to keep the restaurant open.

David Epstein devoted an entire book to the concept of generalists versus specialists in his recently published Range: Why Generalists Triumph in a Specialized World [2]. The book opens with the story of Tiger Woods versus Roger Federer. The classic generalist versus specialist approach to elite status in their sport. At 10 months of age, Tiger Woods was imitating his father's swing with a golf club cut down to his size. By the age of 2, he was driving a golf ball past Bob Hope on National TV. By the age of 4 his father would drop him off at the golf club in the morning and pick him up at night and at age 8, he beat his father for the first time. He continued this singular focus through college into his professional career.

R. W. Wright (✉)
Department of Orthopaedic Surgery, Vanderbilt University Medical Center, Nashville, TN, USA
e-mail: Rick.w.wright@vumc.org

© The Author(s), under exclusive license to Springer Nature Switzerland AG 2022

P. K. Louie et al. (eds.), *The Successful Health Care Professional's Guide*,
https://doi.org/10.1007/978-3-030-95950-0_13

Federer, on the other hand, came to tennis late. His mother was a tennis coach, but his parents never pushed him towards the sport. He played as he said "anything with a ball" growing up. In his teens, he began to gravitate towards tennis, but even then, his parents told him to not take tennis so seriously. He played tennis because it was fun and held himself back from advancing at times to a higher level so that he could keep playing with his friends. Despite the disparate approaches both Tiger and Roger became arguably the best ever at their sport. Which approach was right? It depends somewhat on the activity and the person.

It appears that the activity will reflect whether super specialized practice and early focus to the exclusion of other sports or activities will be beneficial. Repetitive practice appears to benefit those activities where patterns repeat themselves over and over and feedback after each experience improves the next attempt [2]. In domains where there are not repetitive patterns or they are not apparent or feedback is delayed the skill may not be enhanced necessarily through practice. In fact, repetitive training with narrow specialization can result in significantly worse performance when faced by a stressful unknown situation not previously experienced. The person may attempt to use their learned behavior in an inappropriate situation with poor results.

This question has been present for more than 200 years. Adam Smith wrote in the Wealth of Nations in 1776 that specialization was the key to economic advancement for countries [3]. For multiple aspects of life including many professions the decision of generalization versus specialization remains a fundamental decision key to many subsequent decisions and experiences. It may help to define generalist and specialist. According to dictionary.com a generalist is "a person whose knowledge, aptitudes, and skills are applied to the field as a whole or to a variety of different fields" [4]. A specialist "is a person who devotes himself or herself to one subject or to one particular branch of a subject or pursuit". Interestingly a second definition for specialists germane to this discussion is "a medical practitioner who devotes attention to a particular class of diseases, patients, etc." As Konrad Lorenz stated regarding scientists and can be applied to specialists as "people who know more and more about less and less, until they know everything about nothing" [5].

Distinct perceived advantages and disadvantages exist between choosing a pathway of generalization versus specialization. This may be recently evolving. In today's current world, knowledge is the coin of the realm. Generalist's may have a broader based understanding of a variety of topics and people in a variety of fields. Our increasing interconnectedness and ease of communication can make it much easier to solve complex issues utilizing this knowledge and connections. Generalists may have more career flexibility given the broader based knowledge and flexibility that may allow them to be eligible for more opportunities. Jack of all trades, master of none has commonly been used to describe generalists in a negative light, but in reality, the complete original saying was "A jack of all trades is a master of none, but oftentimes better than a master of one" [6]. This changes the entire meaning and illuminates the advantage of a generalist's approach.

Additional advantages for a generalist are their ability to be more global in their approach within organizations and thus frequently assume leadership or managerial positions in companies given the broad skill set. This allows them to more readily navigate uncertainty in the workplace. Disadvantages remain. The increasing breadth of their knowledge requires a sacrifice of depth in any distinct area. Simply having superficial knowledge of a topic may allow you to overlook the nuances that impact dealing with the matter at hand.

Advantages for specialists in addition to the previously recognized potential economic improvements exist. Specialists may gain internal leverage within a company if they represent unique knowledge not otherwise duplicated. This may result in the specialist becoming the true thought leader on a topic within an organization. Disadvantages can include career inflexibility given limited opportunities. You may only be able to find work within this narrow area. With time, companies have melded the two categories and commonly have generalizing-specialists who begin as a generalist but also have depth of knowledge in certain areas [7]. Likewise, a specializing-generalist specializes in a particular field, but has broad understanding of the overall business.

Problem Solving

The domain of problem solving may offer some of the strongest advantages for generalists in a specialist's world. As pointed out by Vikram Mansharamani "Breadth of perspective and the ability to connect the proverbial dots (the domain of generalists) is likely to be as important as depth of expertise and the ability to generate dots (the domain of specialists)" [8]. In medicine we have all been told that "to a person with a hammer everything looks like a nail," but according to Mansharamani if that person had a hammer, a screwdriver and a wrench; might the problem be approached differently with the most effective tool applied to the problem at hand. While being a specialist may not necessarily be a problem, and when a hammer is needed it is useful, it just may be that with more tools the uncertainty of the world around us can be better managed. The only certainty of the future is that it will be uncertain. The broader and more diverse challenges a person has experienced increases their ability to approach a unique new problem.

Medically, you may want to have surgery performed by a specialist working with a familiar team that has worked together multiple times and has predictable outcomes. To solve a new problem or attack a rare condition it may be best to engage a generalist with experience across fields that can contribute to innovative thinking for a new situation.

Additionally, it has been shown that individuals can perform better than teams when solving problems if their experience is diverse. Studies have shown that individuals that have worked across 4 or more genres are better than four individuals teamed together with 4 different expertise domains.

Medical Specialization

How did medical specialization evolve? Or has it always been an aspect of healthcare delivery and only continue to gain attention over the last century. Many forces potentially drove the specialization of medicine. By the end of the 1800s medical knowledge had already grown to the point that it was fundamentally impossible to master it all [9]. Additionally, during this time society in the western world had as a whole slowly evolved towards increasing specialization in skills, labor and knowledge. It would have been unusual for medicine to have resisted the force of this evolution. Academic medicine even in its earliest forms drove this process. Forward thinkers in the medical field began to research and question the approaches in the care of patients and management of diseases. This required individuals to focus on more narrow domains to accumulate the adequate case number to perform this research.

It might be assumed that this inexorable drive occurred consistently across the western world. Paris, France was the modern epicenter of specialization, but in ancient Egypt, specialization in sole body parts was common and Galen wrote that specialization was common in Roman doctors of his time [9]. In Paris, specialists began to enter into their own social category in the 1830s. At this time a specialized eye journal was published 3 times a week for 3 years, and then shortly thereafter, an orthopedic journal was regularly published. From Paris, specialization spread to Vienna, another cultural iconic city of its time. From there, it spread to other North American and European cities with the interesting exception of London.

Specialization was the driver of several other outcomes that are still present today. As George Weisz discusses in The Emergence of Medical Specialization in the Nineteenth Century published in the Bulletin of the History of Medicine in February 2003 [9]. The ability to advance knowledge and also to teach future generations was enhanced by specialists. Professionalism, in the eyes of society, was enhanced by specialization. An appreciation of increased technical knowledge by specialists and increasing technical devices increase the ability to practice a specialized form of medicine. Governmental understanding and support, including support of specialty hospitals, increased credibility. Physicians were still able to combine medical research with private practice which became increasingly lucrative via specialization.

Despite these forces driving specialization there remains significant opposition that seems reminiscent of today's concerns. Generalists remain concerned that super specialization would lose sight of the broader picture of advancing medical knowledge. It also went against a holistic approach to medicine that was common in the era.

London, despite its status as the largest city in Europe lagged the rest of the western world. Several issues contributed to this slower evolution [9]. English practitioners were roughly divided into 3 groups of physicians, surgeons and apothecaries that was slowly in the middle of the nineteenth century evolved into 2 groups of generalists versus elitists. Despite what appeared to be simplification there also existed over 19 licensing bodies with resulting chaos which resulted in a push for simplification versus specialization to gain some order in the field. London also did not have a large dominant teaching hospital that would drive specialization. It was occurring piecemeal at smaller private hospitals, and without that leading entity pushing specialization, specialty development was hampered. Unlike Paris, the medical elite in London were not pursuing research, which also slowed specialization's adoption. In general, while London was a scientific community, it was considered a gentlemanly pursuit of broad knowledge and avoided specialization, even in the Royal Society of London. This reflected the overall academic environment in Britain, where even major universities were not bastions of research advancement. Eventually, in the second half of the nineteenth Century, British physicians recognized the growing role of specialization internationally and it became more common and easier to have a specialist identity within a general hospital. By the early 1900s more than 30% of physicians across Europe identified themselves as a specialist.

Economics

Economic factors enter the equation regarding medical generalists versus specialists. Hsiang et al. in reporting 2017 data collected by a voluntary physician compensation survey conducted by the Medical Group Management Association (MGMA), noted changes following the adoption of the affordable care act. Generalist's (primary care) compensation increased by 1.6% (2.2%) per year, from $214,100 to $247,300 during the period from 2008–2017 [10]. During the same time period specialist's pay from $378,600 to $399,300. Thus, the gap narrowed after ACA adoption. Some issues surrounding this data exist including the fact that MGMA data is not random and there is noted to be overrepresentation of physicians from larger medical groups. Studies have shown that hospital-based physicians or those that are involved in larger systems tend to be compensated at a higher level than those in smaller private practice groups. Additionally, it is expected that specialists would make more given the additional training required and the opportunity costs associated with this additional commitment.

Care Delivery

Ultimately, the most important question is what group provides the best care generalists or specialists? Even this question is fraught with controversy. Is the best care, the cheapest or is it the best outcome? And what outcomes matters most? Patients want timely, easy access, reasonable to low costs, excellent outcomes from providers they like or respect. They may not care if it is a generalist or specialist if these expectations are met. It is inevitable that cost will continue to matter, and the value proposition delivered by a generalist versus a specialist must be considered. In assessing who delivers the best care studies have demonstrated that in the setting of acute myocardial infarction, rheumatoid arthritis, stroke, and asthma; specialists deliver superior outcomes [11]. On the other hand, hypertension, noninsulin dependent diabetes, and low back pain appear to be manage effectively by generalists. Costs can be driven by specialists in a higher direction, and this has been shown in managing low back pain and acute myocardial infarctions. The problem with research in these domains is the inherent biases that cannot be overcome in observational studies. Large database studies do not provide the detail regarding individual patient severity. Specialists may be caring for a more severely affected disease cohort, but this cannot be determined unless a chart review is done on each individual patient which is problematic for any sizable study. The question has relevance as specialists and generalists bicker over patient lives in referrals and managed care settings. This fight for economic life will not go away and will only become more heated as healthcare dollars become scarcer.

The classic example study used to illustrate that specialists do not deliver better care than generalists, is the study evaluating survival rates of acute myocardial infarction during the national cardiologists conference. With thousands of cardiologists not practicing medicine the survival rate actually rose when managed by generalists. This is frequently used to demonstrate that generalist bring a broader more holistic care to the patient and recognize comorbidities and other mitigating factors more readily than a focused specialist [2].

Specialty Choice

Should an individual concern themselves with personality alignment with a specialty choice and if they choose a specialty counterintuitive to their personality will they have career dissatisfaction? This was evaluated by a study assessing residents and a large Midwestern academic Medical Center [12]. This study demonstrated five personality clusters in five broadly defined medical subspecialties. The 5 personality clusters included investigative, commanding, rescuers, dependable, and compassionate. Pathology or internal medicine residents most commonly identified with investigative personality traits. General surgeons were most identified with a commanding personality. Emergency medicine physicians were most commonly identified as rescuers, residents with dependable traits gravitated towards pediatrics, while psychiatry residents demonstrated and identified with compassionate traits most commonly. Interestingly, residents who had traits that were not identified with the most common traits and their specialty actually demonstrated higher life satisfaction scores than those whose traits were consistent with the most common identifying traits in the specialty. Thus, for life satisfaction, choose a specialty that appeals to you even if you are not the classic personality type for that specialty. But, if specializing in any one area gives you a sense of foreboding regarding boredom then choose a generalist approach to medicine specialty choice.

Training

Increasing skill in a multitude of tasks may actually make you better at each one. The skills learned in other settings may improve your ability when tackling a completely different new task. I use this in educating orthopedic residents. I tell them even if you are planning to work in a different subspecialty focusing efforts and maximizing your ability in each specialty both diagnostically and technically will make you a better subspecialist in your ultimate choice.

Well Being

The variety afforded a generalist may benefit their psychological wellbeing. Repeatedly performing the same procedure or dealing with the same diagnoses can lead to boredom and lack of engagement and more recently identified "burnout". While repeatedly performing the same task may improve efficiency initially and overall production at the expense of happiness for the individual. Developing multiple skills can maintain an increased interest in the task at hand. Multiple skills though, does not necessarily mean multitasking which has shown to be inefficient from a production standpoint despite its cultural popularity. Studies have demonstrated that performing multiple tasks over a short amount of time i.e., multitasking decreases happiness. Performing multiple tasks over an extended amount of time improves happiness [2].

Orthopaedics

I am an orthopedic surgeon. I will describe some of the generalist versus specialist issues in the context of orthopedics. The field has undergone tremendous change over the last 50 years. Initially a very generalized specialty there has been increasing forces driving subspecialties. Currently 90% or greater of all orthopedic residency graduates pursue an additional year of training with a subspecialty fellowship [13]. This is represented by the results of our most recent American Academy of Orthopedic Surgeons (AAOS) census data from 2018 published in 2019 [14]. In that census 60% (+/−1.67) of respondents are specialists, 25% (+/−2.29) are general orthopaedic surgeons with specialty interest, and 15% (+/−2.44) are generalists. There are 22 specialty society groups within orthopedics [5]. Thus, well less than 1 in 5 orthopedic surgeons declare themselves to be generalists despite the fact that the average age of practicing orthopedic surgeons is 56.5. So as the field has changed even its older members have sought subspecialty niches within orthopedics.

The results of the AAOS survey will probably not change at any point soon. A relatively recent publication in the Journal of Bone and Joint Surgery (JBJS) reviewing an online survey of 498 residents revealed 91% were planning to pursue a subspecialty fellowship [13]. In the study 430 respondents (86%) were male, 63 (13%) were female. The most popular was sports which 28% planned to pursue. Additional choices included 21%, arthroplasty; 14%, hand surgery, 12%, trauma; 8%, pediatrics; 8%, shoulder and elbow surgery; 8%, spine surgery; 6%, foot and ankle surgery; and 2%, oncology. When queried regarding the reasons for choosing to pursue a fellowship and what type 40% indicated intellectual priorities; 36%, educational; 21%, lifestyle; and 4%, economic. The survey demonstrated women more than men plan to maintain a subspecialty practice (62% versus 34%, respectively, $p < 0.05$).

A concern that must be considered is whether this pursuit of subspecialty training in orthopedics is a surrogate measure of lack of confidence in graduating residents to pursue a generalist practice. This was addressed in a study of Canadian residents [15]. Further development of their surgical skills was considered their most important reason for pursuing additional training. Ability to become employed and future marketability were also rated as important reasons for pursuing fellowship training. Future earnings and malpractice were considered the least important factors. Ninety-four percent believe they were appropriately trained to enter practice after their residency training. Eighty-four percent believed that the current trend in fellowship pursuit did not reflect an inadequacy of training.

A variety of forces have driven this evolution. Orthopedics as a field of knowledge and its procedures has grown exponentially. The ability to remain technically skilled to perform a multitude of procedures in multiple joints and situations has become increasingly challenging. Economic forces have also driven the desire to subspecialized. As our population has become more urban the ability to differentiate themselves within a town of 100+ orthopedic surgeons have rewarded in many areas the subspecialist. Additionally, as residents have chosen to pursue fellowships and emulate their teaching orthopedic surgeons and mentors who are highly specialized; the goal is to hone your skills in a very finite domain as an expert. Specializing and increasing experience with a small number of procedures can be confidence building for patients seeking an expert and can lead to increasing efficiencies and hypothetically decreased complications and improved outcomes. Subspecialists dominate most list of best doctors in any urban setting. However, specializing may lead to physician distribution inequities. The highly specialized surgeon wants a practice in a population center to have enough patients to adequately fill the practice. With increased specialization in orthopedics, it can lead to decreased physicians in rural areas. Economically, increased numbers of specialists can lead to overtreatment and increased medical care utilization. Specializing also exposes the orthopedic surgeon to potential career risk should the field change and demand for a procedure or skill set be eliminated.

However, much like the earlier examples, advantages still exist for the generalist. It can allow you to pursue a more rural lifestyle while still maintaining an adequately busy practice to support you and your family. It can help keep options available when problems are encountered as generalists have been shown to perform better when problem solving. I know that when I attend a general conference that addresses a variety of orthopedic subspecialties, I always leave with new ideas to approach clinical problems and new questions to ask from a clinical research standpoint. A sharing of ideas improves all subspecialties.

The legal aspects of subspecialization can impact the world of orthopedics where malpractice risk remains a real threat for one of the riskiest specialties. The generalist is held to the same standard of care for complex and potentially limb and life-threatening conditions as is the fellowship trained subspecialist. Once you engage upon the care of the patient you are held to the standard of care regardless of your experience or training.

Conclusion

How does a person decide? It ultimately requires insight for the individual. As David Epstein points out in Range, delaying a decision about ultimate career choice, remaining broadly based in experience and education can result in increased happiness and longevity in a career, but we cannot be afraid to change direction when needed as it usually increases satisfaction [2]. With insight, a person will have some understanding as to their personality needs and whether a highly specialized career versus a more general career will remain most interesting for the longest period of time. An understanding of life goals and practice situation can also lend credence to a career decision. Small town rural lifestyles support generalists and urban competitive markets may require a niche or subspecialty approach. All of this is subject to change as outside pressures drive healthcare decisions especially in the form of economics.

References

1. Matteo A. Which is better for your career: specializing or generalizing? 2018; Available from: https://learningenglish.voanews.com/a/which-is-better-for-your-career-specializing-or-generalizing-/4629047.html.
2. Epstein DJ. Range: why generalists triumph in a specialized world. New York: Riverhead Books; 2019. 339 pages
3. Mannino S. Why generalized training can be better than specializing. 2020; Available from: https://www.forbes.com/sites/forbesbusinesscouncil/2020/12/16/why-generalized-training-can-be-better-than-specializing/?sh=782e5d7976f6.
4. 2021; Available from: https://www.dictionary.com/browse/generalist.
5. Bernstein J. Not the last word: specialization and its discontents. Clin Orthop Relat Res. 2015;473(4):1187–8. discussion 1188–91.
6. Wasserman T..; Available from: https://medium.com/@tabithawasserman/the-complete-saying-was-originally-a-jack-of-all-trades-is-a-master-of-none-but-oftentimes-5f4af01a72c6#:~:text=1%20min%20read-,%E2%80%9CThe%20complete%20saying%20was%20originally%20%E2%80%9CA%20jack%20of%20all%20trades,and%20adept%20at%20many%20things.%E2%80%9D.
7. Luenendonk M. The ultimate career choice: generalist vs. specialist. 2019; Available from: https://www.cleverism.com/ultimate-career-choice-generalist-vs-specialist/.
8. Mansharamani, V. Harvard lecturer: 'no specific skill will get you ahead in the future'—but this 'way of thinking' will. 2020; Available from: https://www.cnbc.com/2020/06/15/harvard-yale-researcher-future-success-is-not-a-specific-skill-its-a-type-of-thinking.html.

9. Weisz G. The emergence of medical specialization in the nineteenth century. Bull Hist Med. 2003;77(3):536–75.
10. Hsiang WR, et al. Trends in compensation for primary care and specialist physicians after implementation of the affordable care act. JAMA Netw Open. 2020;3(7):e2011981.
11. Katz JN, Solomon DH, Bates DW. Differences between generalists and specialists. Arthritis Care Res. 1997;10(3):161–2.
12. Sievert M, et al. The influence of temperament and character profiles on specialty choice and well-being in medical residents. PeerJ. 2016;4:e2319.
13. Hariri S, et al. Career plans of current orthopaedic residents with a focus on sex-based and generational differences. J Bone Joint Surg Am. 2011;93(5):e16.
14. Orthopaedic Practice in the US 2018, A.A.o.O. Surgeons, Editor. 2019.
15. Almansoori K, Clark M. Increasing trends in orthopedic fellowships are not due to inadequate residency training. Educat Res Int. 2015;2015:191470. http://dx.doi.org/10.1155/2015/191470.

The Evidence for Diversity

14

Alexandra Arguello and Selina Poon

Definitions

Equality vs Equity

The first step in understanding the evidence for diversity is to recognize the important differences between equality and equity. Many people use these terms interchangeably without understanding how a goal of equality may not fully achieve what it sets out to achieve. In broad terms, equality refers to offering the same opportunities to all, and in healthcare offering equal treatment and resources to all, whereas equity takes into account that not all people start from the same baseline level of opportunity, circumstances, or health [1, 2]. The principle of equity in healthcare aims to distribute resources in a manner than gives everyone what they need in order to reach a common positive outcome. A common illustration of this concept shows three people of varying heights attempting to watch a baseball game from behind a fence. The tall person is able to over the fence, but the average height and shorter person cannot see over the fence. In a situation where equality is the goal, each person would be given one box to stand on, such that now the tall person and average person can see over the fence, but the short person is still unable to see. In a situation where equity is the goal, the tall person does not need the box to see the game so he receives no box, the average person uses one box, and the short person uses two boxes to stand on. All three spectators are now able to see the baseball game over the fence because the resources were allocated preferentially to those who required them to achieve an equal outcome. This is an oversimplification of the concept; however, it is a good way to remember the key differences between equality and equity.

A. Arguello
Department of Orthopedic Surgery, Mayo Clinic, Rochester, MN, USA

S. Poon (✉)
Shriners Childrens Southern California, South Pasadena, CA, USA
e-mail: spoon@shrinenet.org

© The Author(s), under exclusive license to Springer Nature Switzerland AG 2022

P. K. Louie et al. (eds.), *The Successful Health Care Professional's Guide*,
https://doi.org/10.1007/978-3-030-95950-0_14

Justice

Justice is one of the core tenets of medical ethics, which in general is defined as fairness and treating all with equal respect. In medicine, the most prevalent type of justice is distributive justice, which has been defined as the "fair and appropriate distribution of benefits, risks and costs within a society" [3].

Implicit Bias

Implicit bias refers to attitudes and ideas about certain groups of people that can unconsciously affect the way we behave with people who belong to those groups, and in the setting of healthcare, implicit biases can affect the way we interact with and treat diverse patient populations [4]. Although there are proponents and critics of its use and validity, the Harvard Implicit Association Test (IAT) is one of the most common tools used by healthcare professionals and trainees to uncover implicit biases that one may have. A systematic review of implicit biases in healthcare found that most healthcare providers do harbor implicit biases that could potentially affect the way they interact with patients [5].

Inclusion

Many workplaces and healthcare institutions have created departments for diversity and inclusion. While increasing diversity can be understood as efforts to bring someone to the table, if that person is not actively supported or continues feels like an outsider, they will not be able to perform to the best of their abilities. Inclusion is defined as the "process of creating a working culture and environment that recognizes, appreciates, and effectively utilizes the talents, skills, and perspectives of every [team member]; uses team member's skills to achieve the agency's objectives and mission; connects each team member to the organization; and encourages collaboration, flexibility, and fairness" [6]. Diversity and inclusion go hand in hand because even if you have a diverse group of people recruited to a team, if there is no effort put into creating a collaborative and inclusive culture, the group will not live up to its potential.

Cultural Competence vs Cultural Humility

The ever-increasing diversity of the population we serve as healthcare workers in the USA means that we are nearly guaranteed to take care of patients who are culturally different from us. Cultural competence has been defined as a "means of attending to the culturally diverse backgrounds of patients, providing person-centered care, and reducing health disparities" [7]. Culturally competent health care is the goal of many workshops and training sessions for medical students and residents alike. While the concept and definition of cultural competence are well-intentioned, the issue with it stems from the implication that you can become fully proficient in understanding the intricacies of countless groups of people and has been referred to as a "static goal" [4, 7]. If a person feels they have achieved cultural competence, they are closing themselves off to the possibility of life-long learning and likely stereotyping patients based on incomplete understanding. There has been a call to shift from the term cultural competence to cultural humility, which has also been referred to as cultural sensitivity or cultural curiosity [4, 7, 8]. Rather than working to increase your knowledge base regarding individual cultures, the process of cultural humility works toward "admit(ting) one does not know and (becoming) willing to learn from patients about their experiences, while being aware of one's own embeddedness in culture(s)" [7]. Specifically, cultural humility training focuses more on actively listening to the individual patient and participating in self-reflection to ensure biases and stereotypes are not affecting the physician's ability to provide excellent care to that patient [8].

Structural Racism

Structural racism has been defined as "the totality of ways in which societies foster racial discrimination, through mutually reinforcing inequitable systems (in housing, education, employment, earnings, benefits, credit, media, health care, criminal justice, and so on) that in turn reinforce discriminatory beliefs, values, and distribution of resources, which together affect the risk of adverse health outcomes" [9]. Although socioeconomic status is commonly referred to as a significant cause of health inequities, Phelan and Link reported that racism is the "ultimate target" that has to be eliminated in order to move toward health equity amongst all races [10]. One example of structural racism and its effect on health inequities is residential segregation, also known as redlining [11, 12]. This Home Owners' Loan Corporation (HOLC) governmental policy from the 1930s resulted in racial disparities in mortgage lending in different residential areas, resulting in a majority of mortgage loan approvals going to predominantly white residents rather than people of color [13]. Since then, residential segregation has continued to foster disparities in homeownership, education, and access to healthcare. Residential segregation has recently been linked to health disparities in hypertension, breast cancer, preterm birth, and asthma [12–15].

Why Diversity Is Important in General

In his 2016 memorandum regarding promoting diversity, President Obama wrote "diverse groups are more effective at problem solving than homogeneous groups, and policies that promote diversity and inclusion will enhance our ability to draw from the broadest possible pool of talent, solve our toughest challenges, maximize employee engagement and innovation, and lead by example by setting a high standard for providing access to opportunity to all segments of our society" [16]. When diversity is valued and fostered, it is associated with increased innovation within companies and increased productivity [17]. Although it may feel more comfortable to work with people who are similar to you, different perspectives, backgrounds, experiences, and attitudes that a diverse workforce fosters has repeatedly been shown to have superior results [18].

The McKinsey & Company report *Diversity Matters* defined diversity as "a greater share of women and a more mixed ethnic/racial composition in the leadership of large companies" when they sought to measure the relationship between diversity with financial performance on a global level [19]. The data from hundreds of companies in the UK, US, Latin America, and Canada revealed that companies with the most racial/ethnic diversity and gender diversity were 35% and 15% more likely, respectively, to be more financially profitable. Although this represents a correlation rather than causation, they go on to describe how diversity positively impacts companies including the ability to relate to the customer base and increased employee satisfaction.

Healthcare

Patient Outcomes

A large body of research exists that highlights the importance of diversity in healthcare settings as it relates to patient outcomes [17, 20–22]. A survey of over 92,000 patients found that patients reported a more positive healthcare experience when they were treated by physicians who share their race/ethnicity [21]. They concluded with idea that "efforts to improve the physician workforce diversity are imperative" [21]. When patients have a more positive experience with their healthcare provider, they are much more likely to trust their physician, adhere to treatment plans, and return for follow-up visits. Although it may not be feasible to always match each patient with a physician whose background is concordant with their own, the current demographic of the physician workforce does not represent the demographic of the population they serve.

There have been countless examples of health inequities that occur among racial minorities [23]. Because of the abundant literature that has shown Black patients are significantly less likely to receive adequate pain control when compared to white patients [24–26], non-medically trained white people as well as white medical students and residents were surveyed regarding misconceptions about biological differences between races [27]. Both of these groups endorsed untrue beliefs including the myth that Black people's "skin is thicker than whites'" and that Black people have "less sensitive nerve endings" compared to white people [27]. This article shines light upon the idea that the meaning of race is confused with genetics in medicine, and that racism is ingrained into medical education. In medical school, we are all taught to memorize that the equation for estimated glomerular filtration rate for Black patients is different than any other race, resulting in reported "better kidney function" for Black patients with the same blood creatinine level as white patients. This is a detail that is integrated into the electronic medical record, yet recently this "race-corrected" equation is a topic of controversy, with one side arguing that race is a social construct rather than a biological construct and the other arguing that there is a biological basis to the equation that will result in overdiagnosis and overtreatment if it is not utilized [28, 29]. Similar "race corrections" exist in multiple medical specialties including cardiology, obstetrics, and urology, many times without adequate data to support the algorithms [28]. Overall, the idea of race being a social construct rather than a biological construct is a reminder for clinicians to take the totality of the patient into account when treating them. Understanding and awareness of the detrimental effect of structural racism, opportunity gaps, and health inequities is critical to moving forward with the mindset of doing all possible to mitigate these and taking care of patients in an equitable and evidence-based manner. A diverse workforce is better equipped to take these complexities into account and work toward health equity.

Training Experience

As a healthcare student and trainee, you learn from your peers, professors, more senior trainees, attendings, and other healthcare providers. A survey of over 600 medical students reported that a majority of the students found that racial and ethnic diversity among their medical school peers enhanced their education and their experiences [30]. Over half of the respondents felt that diversity in the medical school setting would lead to "alternative viewpoints being seriously discussed," which mirrors the sentiment that diverse groups of people bring with them life experiences and viewpoints that enhance the environment. Further, an analysis of the 2007–2018 NRMP Applicant Survey from the residency match process found that applicants across specialties are increasingly taking "geographic and institutional diversity" into account when applying and creating their rank lists [31]. These studies reflect the increasing awareness from students and trainees that a diverse environment is necessary for expanding one's cultural humility and should be prioritized.

Where Is Orthopaedics Now? (The Field That I Currently Work In)

A survey of program directors and coordinators aimed to elucidate the perceived barriers to improving diversity in orthopaedic surgery residency programs [32]. In an analysis of ten cycles of residency match data, with academic data taken into account, Asian, Black, Hispanic, and "Other" races were associated with a lower odds of matching into an orthopaedic surgery residency [33]. Currently, the orthopaedic workforce is the least diverse of all medical specialties, where women make up 15% of orthopaedic surgery residents, 4.1% are Black, and 2.7% are Hispanic [34, 35]. Without a concerted effort to increase diversity in orthopaedic surgery, a recent study suggested it would take until the year 2354 to reach 50% women in orthopaedic surgery [36].

How Trainees Can Help/Participate

As Mentors

A mentor-mentee relationship is crucial for making students feel like they belong in a certain field when they may not see many people that look like them or come from a similar background. A survey of over 4800 members of the American Association of Cardiology in 2020 found that mentees whose gender identity or race/ethnicity was concordant with those of their mentors reported positive outcomes from the mentorship relationship [37]. They drew the conclusion that it is important for more female and underrepresented minority cardiologists to volunteer their time and energy to mentor trainees or medical students. Importantly, they note that they "are not discounting the benefits that can be derived from cross-sex or cross-ethnicity mentoring relationships" [37]. In specialties such as orthopaedic surgery where the percentage of female and URM surgeons is miniscule, it is imperative that the responsibility of increasing diversity does not fall solely on those who fit in those categories. This concept has been referred to as the "minority tax" or more recently "Underrepresented Minority in Medicine faculty responsibility disparity" [38]. The burden of initiatives to increase diversity falls on URM and female faculty and many of those responsibilities are intangibles that will not support their promotion. This in turn furthers the disparities in the diversity of leadership because there are fewer women and URM faculty achieving academic promotion to the professor level and into leadership positions. Even if you do not find yourself in one of these minority groups, you should still take an active role in diversity and inclusion initiatives, mentoring to the best of your abilities, and lightening the load of your diverse colleagues who may need assistance with the recruitment and mentorship initiatives.

Mentorship and sponsorship are concepts that have many overlapping responsibilities, but in the discussion of diversity and inclusion, sponsorship tends to become more important [39]. Where a mentor is typically someone who can offer advice, provide feedback, and help mentees develop professionally and personally, sponsorship involves providing tangibles that can lead to career advancement. Sponsorship has been reported to be especially important for women and underrepresented minorities in medicine [39–41]. It is well documented that there are gender disparities in physician wages across all medical specialties, and there are also disparities in academic promotion of women and URM's [42, 43]. An excerpt from the Harvard Business Review presents some of the specific actions of a sponsor which include visibly and vocally advocating for the person being sponsored, facilitating connections and networking opportunities with senior leaders, and actively presents career opportunities [44]. In the academic medicine world, some other examples could include offering collaboration on various research initiatives or nominating for speaking opportunities at conferences and to national societies to promote visibility. Even as trainees, you have more influence than you realize. Reflect upon the research and or quality improvement projects where you have the ability to invite different members to the team. Suggest different topic and speakers to enhance your overall learning in addition to your specialty training with special consideration to have adequate representation of the diversity.

As Bystanders/Upstanders

As a healthcare professional, you are held to a high moral standard and in general the public trusts you to do the right thing. In situations where you are witness to discrimination, bias, or harassment based on gender identity, race, sexual orientation, language, religion, or any other personal quality, your response as an active bystander can make a difference. Bystander intervention training typically includes the "5 D's" (Fig. 14.1) available online courtesy of the Hollaback! Organization [45]. **Direct** refers to directly letting the perpetrator know that they are doing something that is harmful or inappropriate, either with verbal or non-verbal methods. This can include shaking your head to express your concern or directly asking the person to clarify what they were trying to express. The phrase "do you mind clarifying what you mean by that statement?" is likely to cause the perpetrator to be introspective and potentially apologize to the victim. The second D, **Distract,** involves methods such as changing the topic of discussion or bringing attention to something else in the room. **Delegate** means to escalate the issue to someone more senior, perhaps an attending or administrator if it is happening amongst colleagues in the hospital. **Delay** refers to following up with the victim after the event has occurred to show support. Finally, **document** highlights the importance of documenting a

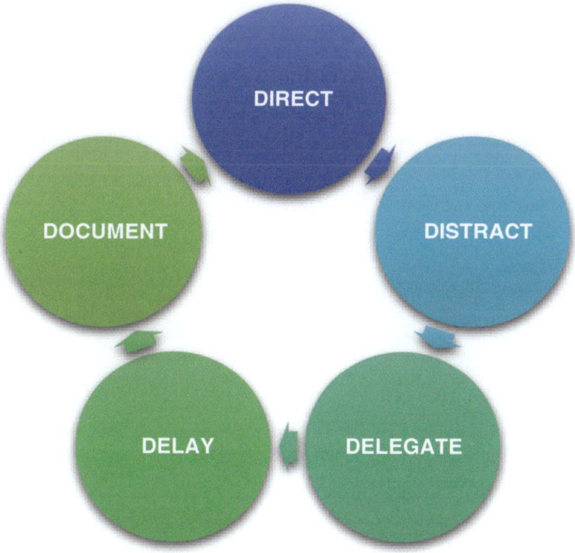

Fig. 14.1 The "5D's" of bystander intervention training. (Modified with permission from Julie B. Samora, MD)

situation by way of taking notes or possibly audio or video recording an event if someone else is already aiding the victim.

Another phrase to be aware of that falls under the umbrella of serving as an ally for someone who may be discriminated against or harassed in your presence is acting as an upstander [46]. In contrast to a passive bystander who observes an event take place, an upstander has been defined as "a person who intervenes or acts in support of an individual who is being attacked or bullied" [46]. Wheeler et al. described an unfortunately common scenario in which a member of the healthcare team is harassed, discriminated against, or subject to microaggressions by patients or their families, and this is an ideal scenario for trainees to serve as an upstander and de-escalate the situation [47]. The authors describe 12 recommendations for addressing that type of situation. Perhaps the most applicable of these is Tip #3, which walks the reader through determining whether to respond to the offender at the time of the altercation. These situations can arise at times where it would be inappropriate to immediately respond, such as if some form of immediate medical attention was necessary due to an emergency [48]. If there is no obvious barrier to addressing the situation, the next step is to "check your own reaction [47]," meaning discrimination and hateful words can cause an innate response even if they are not directed at you. Wheeler et al. describes the activation of the sympathetic nervous system as something that can hinder an upstander's ability to analyze and respond to the situation appropriately and in a way that will be productive. The authors caution that although it is natural to feel uncomfortable when witnessing an injustice occur, this should not hinder you from responding to the offender.

Social Media

It is common for students to choose a specialty because they had a mentor or role model who helped them along the way. Sometimes students do not have access to those mentors or role models at their home institutions, so another way for trainees to influence the pool of applicants and act as a mentor is to be an active participant on social media to connect with potential applicants. Social media became an important resource for applicants during the COVID-19 pandemic, where applicants used various platforms to interact with residents and learn more about the culture of residency programs [49]. As a trainee, you can make yourself available to virtually meet with students to discuss their applications, answer questions, and guide them during the residency process.

Social media can be both beneficial and detrimental during your medical career. It can be used as an avenue to connect with your patients, and this is something to keep in mind as you enter your career as a healthcare professional. A recent study analyzing Twitter content posted by healthcare professionals utilized software that was able to access tweets that had been deleted by the author, which serves as a reminder that everything posted to the internet is permanent [50].

Continued Learning in Practice

Because the topic of diversity is ever-changing and at times controversial, it is of the utmost importance to stay current in the literature and understand that it is a lifelong learning process. The most effective allies are those who are consistently aware of their own actions and biases and are aware of their surroundings and any injustices that need to be addressed. The more frequently you put yourself in situations to be an ally, the more comfortable you will become.

Mitigating unconscious bias is another aspect of continued learning and actively working to create a better environment for your colleagues and your patients. Marcelin et al. listed common strategies that are used to mitigate unconscious bias at the individual and organizational level [4]. Frequent introspection on your personal biases, continually working toward cultural humility, and participating in mentorship and sponsorship are some such strategies. At the organizational level, some strategies include diversity and inclusion training that is validated and meaningful and ensuring there is a commitment to a culture of inclusivity from the top down. Like most of the other strategies already discussed, mitigating unconscious bias is a goal that cannot be completed, but must be consistently worked toward.

The *Her Time is Now* Report spearheaded by Dr. Julie Silver is a comprehensive resource that highlights the issues with lack of diversity in healthcare and details methods that various healthcare leaders have used to improve the diversity and inclusion at their institutions [43]. The topics highlighted in this resource include the importance of closing the gender pay gap, improving the vast disparities in the gender makeup of the governing societies of each medical specialty, including women in expert panels and speaking opportunities, being ethical in the distribution of funding and grant money, and being equitable in academic promotion.

The importance of and benefits of diversity demonstrated in the literature are robust. One of the most effective ways to make a difference in this domain as you go through training and then continue to climb the academic ladder is to extend a hand to those behind you and lift them as you climb. In order to positively influence the diversification of your specialty, pay special attention to those who are underrepresented and who may not have access to the resources and opportunities that others are afforded when deciding who you are going to mentor and sponsor. Becoming involved in different organizations and outreach/pipeline programs to act as a mentor is an impactful way to connect with underrepresented students, including Nth Dimensions [51] and the Perry Initiative [52], both of which have been successful in the recruitment of URM students. Further, organizations such as the Ruth Jackson Orthopaedic Society, the J. Robert Gladden Orthopaedic Society, and the American Association for Latino Orthopaedic Surgeons are organizations aimed at actively working to increase diversity and inclusion in the field of orthopaedic surgery.

References

1. Machado FR. All in a day's work—equity vs. equality at a public ICU in Brazil. N Engl J Med. 2016;375(25):2420–1.
2. George Washington University oMoPHp. Equity vs. Equality: What's the Difference? https://onlinepublichealth.gwu.edu/resources/equity-vs-equality/2020.
3. Fisher OM, Brown KGM, Coker DJ, McBride KE, Steffens D, Koh CE, et al. Distributive justice during the coronavirus disease 2019 pandemic in Australia. ANZ J Surg. 2020;90(6):961–2.
4. Marcelin JR, Siraj DS, Victor R, Kotadia S, Maldonado YA. The impact of unconscious bias in healthcare: how to recognize and mitigate it. J Infect Dis. 2019;220(220 Suppl 2):S62–s73.
5. Hall WJ, Chapman MV, Lee KM, Merino YM, Thomas TW, Payne BK, et al. Implicit racial/ethnic bias among health care professionals and its influence on health care outcomes: a systematic review. Am J Public Health. 2015;105(12):e60–76.
6. Diversity and Inclusion Definitions. https://www.hud.gov/program_offices/administration/admabout/diversity_inclusion/definitions.
7. Lekas HM, Pahl K, Fuller LC. Rethinking cultural competence: shifting to cultural humility. Health Serv Insights. 2020;13:1178632920970580.
8. Sprik P, Gentile D. Cultural humility: a way to reduce LGBTQ health disparities at the end of life. Am J Hosp Palliat Care. 2020;37(6):404–8.
9. Bailey ZD, Krieger N, Agénor M, Graves J, Linos N, Bassett MT. Structural racism and health inequities in the USA: evidence and interventions. Lancet. 2017;389(10077):1453–63.
10. Phelan JC, Link BG. Is racism a fundamental cause of inequalities in health? Annu Rev Sociol. 2015;41:311–30.
11. Riley AR. Neighborhood disadvantage, residential segregation, and beyond—lessons for studying structural racism and health. J Racial Ethn Health Disparities. 2018;5(2):357–65.
12. Kershaw KN, Diez Roux AV, Burgard SA, Lisabeth LD, Mujahid MS, Schulz AJ. Metropolitan-level racial residential segregation and black-white disparities in hypertension. Am J Epidemiol. 2011;174(5):537–45.
13. Krieger N, Van Wye G, Huynh M, Waterman PD, Maduro G, Li W, et al. Structural racism, historical redlining, and risk of preterm birth in New York City, 2013–2017. Am J Public Health. 2020;110(7):1046–53.
14. Collin LJ, Gaglioti AH, Beyer KM, Zhou Y, Moore MA, Nash R, et al. Neighborhood-level redlining and lending bias are associated with breast cancer mortality in a large and diverse metropolitan area. Cancer Epidemiol Biomark Prev. 2021;30(1):53–60.
15. Nardone A, Casey JA, Morello-Frosch R, Mujahid M, Balmes JR, Thakur N. Associations between historical residential redlining and current age-adjusted rates of emergency department visits due to asthma across eight cities in California: an ecological study. Lancet Planet Health. 2020;4(1):e24–31.
16. Obama B. Presidential Memorandum. Promoting Diversity and Inclusion in the National Security Workforce, 05.10. 2016. Washington, DC: The White House 2016. Online: whitehouse.gov (archives.gov). 2018;21.
17. Gomez LE, Bernet P. Diversity improves performance and outcomes. J Natl Med Assoc. 2019;111(4):383–92.
18. Rock D, Grant H. Why diverse teams are smarter. Harv Bus Rev. 2016;4(4):2–5.
19. Hunt V, Layton D, Prince S. Diversity matters. McKinsey & Company. 2015;1(1):15–29.
20. Hilton EJ, Lunardi N, Sreedharan R, Goff KL, Batakji M, Rosenberger DS. Two sides of the same coin: addressing racial and gender disparities among physicians and the impact on the community they serve. Anesthesiol Clin. 2020;38(2):369–77.
21. Takeshita J, Wang S, Loren AW, Mitra N, Shults J, Shin DB, et al. Association of Racial/ethnic and gender concordance between patients and physicians with patient experience ratings. JAMA Netw Open. 2020;3(11):e2024583.
22. Reede JY. A recurring theme: the need for minority physicians. Health Aff (Millwood). 2003;22(4):91–3.

23. Gee GC, Ford CL. Structural racism and health inequities: old issues, new directions. Du Bois Rev. 2011;8(1):115–32.
24. Cintron A, Morrison RS. Pain and ethnicity in the United States: a systematic review. J Palliat Med. 2006;9(6):1454–73.
25. Todd KH, Deaton C, D'Adamo AP, Goe L. Ethnicity and analgesic practice. Ann Emerg Med. 2000;35(1):11–6.
26. Shavers VL, Bakos A, Sheppard VB. Race, ethnicity, and pain among the U.S. adult population. J Health Care Poor Underserved. 2010;21(1):177–220.
27. Hoffman KM, Trawalter S, Axt JR, Oliver MN. Racial bias in pain assessment and treatment recommendations, and false beliefs about biological differences between blacks and whites. Proc Natl Acad Sci U S A. 2016;113(16):4296–301.
28. Vyas DA, Eisenstein LG, Jones DS. Hidden in plain sight – reconsidering the use of race correction in clinical algorithms. N Engl J Med. 2020;383(9):874–82.
29. Eneanya ND, Yang W, Reese PP. Reconsidering the consequences of using race to estimate kidney function. JAMA. 2019;322(2):113–4.
30. Whitla DK, Orfield G, Silen W, Teperow C, Howard C, Reede J. Educational benefits of diversity in medical school: a survey of students. Acad Med. 2003;78(5):460–6.
31. Dinh JV, Salas E. Prioritization of diversity during the residency match: trends for a new workforce. J Grad Med Educ. 2019;11(3):319–23.
32. McDonald TC, Drake LC, Replogle WH, Graves ML, Brooks JT. Barriers to increasing diversity in orthopaedics: the residency program perspective. JB JS Open Access. 2020;5(2):e0007.
33. Poon SC, Nellans K, Gorroochurn P, Chahine NO. Race, but not gender, is associated with admissions into orthopaedic residency programs. Clin Orthop Relat Res. 2020. https://doi.org/10.1097/CORR.0000000000001553. Epub ahead of print. PMID: 33229901.
34. Day MA, Owens JM, Caldwell LS. Breaking barriers: a brief overview of diversity in orthopedic surgery. Iowa Orthop J. 2019;39(1):1–5.
35. Poon S, Kiridly D, Mutawakkil M, Wendolowski S, Gecelter R, Kline M, et al. Current trends in sex, race, and ethnic diversity in orthopaedic surgery residency. J Am Acad Orthop Surg. 2019;27(16):e725–e33.
36. Acuña AJ, Sato EH, Jella TK, Samuel LT, Jeong SH, Chen AF, et al. How long will it take to reach gender parity in orthopaedic surgery in the United States? An analysis of the national provider identifier registry. Clin Orthop Relat Res. 2021;479:1179–89.
37. Abudayyeh I, Tandon A, Wittekind SG, Rzeszut AK, Sivaram CA, Freeman AM, et al. Landscape of mentorship and its effects on success in cardiology. JACC Basic Transl Sci. 2020;5(12):1181–6.
38. Rodríguez JE, Campbell KM, Pololi LH. Addressing disparities in academic medicine: what of the minority tax? BMC Med Educ. 2015;15:6.
39. Ayyala MS, Skarupski K, Bodurtha JN, González-Fernández M, Ishii LE, Fivush B, et al. Mentorship is not enough: exploring sponsorship and its role in career advancement in academic medicine. Acad Med. 2019;94(1):94–100.
40. Travis EL, Doty L, Helitzer DL. Sponsorship: a path to the academic medicine C-suite for women faculty? Acad Med. 2013;88(10):1414–7.
41. Gottlieb AS, Travis EL. Rationale and models for career advancement sponsorship in academic medicine: the time is here; the time is now. Acad Med. 2018;93(11):1620–3.
42. Warner AS, Lehmann LS. Gender wage disparities in medicine: time to close the gap. J Gen Intern Med. 2019;34(7):1334–6.
43. Her Time is Now Version 2. https://sheleadshealthcare.com/wp-content/uploads/2020/09/HerTimeIsNow_Report.pdf; 2020.
44. Hewlett SA, Peraino K, Sherbin L, Sumberg K. The sponsor effect: breaking through the last glass ceiling. Boston: Harvard Business Review; 2010.
45. Guide to Bystander Training. https://www.ihollaback.org/guide-bystander-intervention/
46. Ho CP, Chong A, Narayan A, Cooke EA, Deng F, Agarwal V, et al. Mitigating Asian American bias and xenophobia in response to the coronavirus pandemic: how you can be an Upstander. J Am Coll Radiol. 2020;17(12):1692–4.

47. Wheeler DJ, Zapata J, Davis D, Chou C. Twelve tips for responding to microaggressions and overt discrimination: when the patient offends the learner. Med Teach. 2019;41(10):1112–7.
48. Whitgob EE, Blankenburg RL, Bogetz AL. The Discriminatory Patient and Family: Strategies to Address Discrimination Towards Trainees. Acad Med. 2016;91(11 Association of American Medical Colleges Learn Serve Lead: Proceedings of the 55th Annual Research in Medical Education Sessions):S64-s9.
49. Goshtasbi K, Tsutsumi K, Berger MH, Kuan EC, Tjoa T, Haidar YM. Otolaryngology residency programs' rising social media presence during the COVID-19 pandemic. Laryngoscope. 2021;131(5):E1457–e9.
50. Ahmed W, Jagsi R, Gutheil TG, Katz MS. Public disclosure on social media of identifiable patient information by health professionals: content analysis of twitter data. J Med Internet Res. 2020;22(9):e19746.
51. Mason BS, Ross W, Chambers MC, Grant R, Parks M. Pipeline program recruits and retains women and underrepresented minorities in procedure based specialties: a brief report. Am J Surg. 2017;213(4):662–5.
52. Lattanza LL, Meszaros-Dearolf L, O'Connor MI, Ladd A, Bucha A, Trauth-Nare A, et al. The Perry Initiative's medical student outreach program recruits women into orthopaedic residency. Clin Orthop Relat Res. 2016;474(9):1962–6.

Correction to: The Successful Health Care Professional's Guide

Philip K. Louie, Michael H. McCarthy, and Todd J. Albert

Correction to:
Philip K. Louie Michael H. McCarthy Todd J. Albert (eds.),
The Successful Health Care Professional's Guide,
https://doi.org/10.1007/978-3-030-95950-0

This book was inadvertently published with incorrect affiliation of the editor Michael H. McCarthy which has now been corrected as follows:

"Michael H. McCarthy, Indiana Spine Group, University of Indiana, Carmel, IN, USA".

The updated version of the book can be found at
https://doi.org/10.1007/978-3-030-95950-0

© The Author(s), under exclusive license to Springer Nature Switzerland AG 2022
P. K. Louie et al. (eds.), *The Successful Health Care Professional's Guide*,
https://doi.org/10.1007/978-3-030-95950-0_15

Index

© The Author(s), under exclusive license to Springer Nature Switzerland AG 2022
P. K. Louie et al. (eds.), *The Successful Health Care Professional's Guide*,
https://doi.org/10.1007/978-3-030-95950-0

MIX
Papier aus verantwortungsvollen Quellen
Paper from responsible sources
FSC® C105338

If you have any concerns about our products,
you can contact us on
ProductSafety@springernature.com

In case Publisher is established outside the EU,
the EU authorized representative is:
Springer Nature Customer Service Center GmbH
Europaplatz 3, 69115 Heidelberg, Germany

Printed by Libri Plureos GmbH
in Hamburg, Germany